GENERATION ANXIETY

Dr. Lauren Cook

GENERATION ANXIETY

A MILLENNIAL AND GEN Z GUIDE TO STAYING AFLOAT IN AN UNCERTAIN WORLD

ABRAMS IMAGE, NEW YORK

Editor: Soyolmaa Lkhagvadorj
Designer: Danielle Youngsmith
Managing Editor: Glenn Ramirez
Production Manager: Larry Pekarek

Library of Congress Control Number: 2023933936

ISBN: 978-1-4197-6801-9
eISBN: 979-8-88707-022-3

Printed and bound in the United States

10 9 8 7 6 5 4 3 2 1

Abrams Image books are available at special discounts when purchased in
quantity for premiums and promotions as well as fundraising or educational
use. Special editions can also be created to specification. For details, contact
specialsales@abramsbooks.com or the address below.

Abrams Image® is a registered trademark of Harry N. Abrams, Inc.

ABRAMS The Art of Books
195 Broadway, New York, NY 10007
abramsbooks.com

To Greg:
This too shall pass . . . and that's why I don't want
to miss a moment of this life with you.

To my new son, Derek:
I'm so glad that I didn't let my anxiety stop me from living out the
most incredible adventure by welcoming you into the world.

And to my Siamese cat, Mochi:
Because more books should be dedicated to our pets, as they're
the ultimate antidote for our anxiety. Mochi is no exception.

CONTENTS

INTRODUCTION

IF YOU FEEL LIKE YOU'RE DROWNING, IT'S NOT JUST YOU

"Jack. Jack! There's a boat." We all know that famous scene at the end of *Titanic* when Kate Winslet is staring at a freezing Leonardo DiCaprio after the unsinkable boat has indeed sunk. As Rose (played by Winslet) lies belly-down across the length of the door in her life jacket, we see Jack clinging to the side with just his head afloat. By the time the lifeboat comes by, Rose realizes that it's too late and she has to let Jack go into the frigid abyss.

What really has become meme-worthy today, though, is the realization that the doorframe Kate Winslet was lying on was definitely big enough for the two of them. While Rose stayed warmish on that big block of cedar, her newfound love had to cling to the side, Mufasa-style, before the wildebeests came.[1]

Many of us can relate to Rose and Jack. Chances are, you're picking up this book because you're fed up with your anxiety. Whether you're Rose, too paralyzed to take action, or you're Jack and you feel like you're barely clinging on, this book is meant to be the life jacket that can buoy you to give you the support you need. You don't have to shiver in the water anymore. As a psychologist with a doctorate in clinical psychology and a master's in marriage and family therapy (and really just as a human being), I get it. I live with anxiety myself. I treat my clients' anxiety on a daily basis and I've seen intimately how challenging (and underrated) anxiety can be.

People often talk about anxiety like it's low-hanging fruit. "Doesn't everyone have anxiety now?" "Isn't something wrong with you if you *don't* have anxiety?" When I hear comments like these, I know it's a sign of a gap between a judgment call and the actual lived experience. Because for those who do live with anxiety, it's no small beast. I think most of us would choose to live anxiety-free if we could.

It's clear to me that we're all seeking help for our anxiety—look no further than TikTok and Instagram and you'll see #mentalhealthmatters trending much of the time (and not just during Mental Health Awareness Month in May). When I started posting on my TikTok to shed light on common disorders such as anxiety, panic attacks, and anxious attachment, I had no idea there would be more than two hundred thousand followers trying to better understand why they were struggling and what they could do about it. It's not that I had the best dance moves (trust me, you can go look for yourself) or that I did great outfits of the day (though I do wear some pretty fun, colorful dresses if I do say so myself). People just genuinely want to feel better, and accessible platforms such as TikTok provide a quick way to get the conversation started.

So, if you ever feel like you're battling your anxiety alone, let me assure you that you definitely aren't. In fact, if you're one of the 40 million Americans who experience clinical anxiety, welcome to the club you likely didn't want to be invited to. I'm going to be telling you some hard truths—but I'm also going to give you some welcome answers to start and stay feeling better.

As you'll soon see, I find that honesty is the best policy, especially when it comes to anxiety. I'm sure I could tell you many things you'd love to hear instead. I could tell you that I have the magic wand to make your anxiety go away. I could tell you that I have the ticket that's going to get you out of this awful place where your stomach churns and your heart races all the time. Many people have made millions of dollars selling you this fantasy, and we have gladly paid because we'll do anything to not feel uncomfortable or unsafe.

But as you'll soon see in this book, my stance is different. I'm not here to bestow a magic spell on you. I'm not here to "fix" you or "change" you. And the wild thing is, it's in this *not* trying to fix or change how you feel—when you simply allow the anxiety to be there—that you may actually start to feel better. It's in this notion of dropping the rope, riding the wave, and letting it *be* that you may see anxiety loosen its grip over you. Hard to believe?

If you're skeptical, I get it. We've been socialized to believe that anytime something is uncomfortable, we should try to cut it out or make it go away. So why wouldn't we try to do that with anxiety, right? Wouldn't we want to have as little anxiety as possible?

Not necessarily. A little anxiety can be the impetus to our caring. It can give us that surge of energy to study for the exam we've been procrastinating on all month. It can be the bell that rings, telling us it's time to stand up for ourselves when someone is taking advantage of us. But even if we wanted to make anxiety go away, we really couldn't. And in reality, something would be a little off with our brains if we didn't have an appropriate fear response.

Take for example the *Free Solo* documentary featuring Alex Honnold, where he climbs the three-thousand-foot vertical rock face of El Capitan without a single rope. If you've watched this like I did and didn't breathe for an hour and a half as your eyes were glued to the screen, this is a sign of a normal responding brain that has an appropriate fear response (thank you, mirror neurons that make you feel what others are feeling, including through a screen). We learn that Honnold's amygdala, or fear center of his brain, has a much lower activation level than the average person's. It's likely because of this difference in neurology that he can do such a feat without having a full-blown meltdown every step of the way.

So, unless you wish that you too could free-climb in Yosemite, anxiety is your brain's way of trying to look out for you. The problem is that, for many of us, we have the opposite problem that Honnold has. Our amygdala is *overly* activated. Whereas the average person would startle at a snake, we startle at a snake, a bunny, and even an inanimate doll or two (but let's be real—those can be just as creepy as a snake if you ask me). This is why many of us have a love-hate relationship with our anxiety. While we hate the way it makes us feel, both physically and emotionally, we also tend to have a deep-rooted belief that it's protecting us, and we'd feel guilty if we let our anxiety go. After all, don't we owe everything—our success, our security, our (in)sanity—to it?

That's why changing your relationship with anxiety is going to take some willingness on your part. This is especially challenging if you've learned to cling to doubt and mistrust as defense mechanisms to keep you from getting hurt. But I want you to imagine me standing behind you, reminding you it's okay to fall. It's okay to feel a little exposed. I've got your back.

You may be stiffening up already. I understand why you're tense— why you feel like you have to have the checking, organizing, people-pleasing, controlling, and maybe even manipulating behavior in place. It's your way to feel protected in a very unsafe world. The problem is that the more we use these devices, the more out of control and anxious we feel.

We often feel like we need these behaviors to prevent any possible pain in our lives. If you've been using this strategy, though, then you know how utterly exhausting this is. Remembering to check "just one more time," asking your loved ones to reassure you, and wondering whether it will all be okay is like putting your brain through a car chase where the tires blow out but you're still trying to escape. One way or another, those fears are always nipping at your heels. You can see how this quickly turns into a vicious cycle where we feel like life is one epic tornado and we are just completely swept up in it.

So, if you're at that point, where you've been in the midst of the storm for some time, this book is going to help you get through it. No, it's not going to save you. But that's the point. I'm going to help you work through the reality that life is going to be hard and scary. We're going to sit with the fact that, ultimately, none of us get out of this thing alive. You may get angry at the audacity of my bluntness, but last time I checked, it's true. The sooner we can sit with this reality, the sooner we can get to liberated living, where we exist in gratitude, rather than fear, for what the day may bring.

As you can see, I like to give it to you straight (but sincerely). Hopefully, that will be refreshing, as I'm sure you've heard enough platitudes at this point, that "everything happens for a reason" or that "there's nothing to be afraid of." As someone who used to dole out those winning one-liners myself, I've seen what works and what doesn't.

The reality is that some things in life don't make any sense. And yes, there's plenty in life to be afraid of. Life is unfair. It's brutal. It's chock-full of nonstop unpredictable events.

Given all this, I get why you're anxious. You hear tragic tales constantly in the news and from friends, and you've likely lived through some in your own life. That doesn't even include the countless narratives your mind has concocted for the future.

We have a key choice when it comes to these experiences, both the lived and the imaginary. We can choose to expend our energy trying to run away from existing heartbreaks and avoiding potential future disasters with fervor . . . or we can accept them for what they are.

We can acknowledge the beautiful and broken reality that life is. We can surrender to the truth that life is indeed unpredictable and sometimes painful. There is incredible power in this perspective. It is in this facing of the truth that we no longer live in the shadow of fear. When we can sit with the reality of life, the gnawing of potential pain no longer owns us.

Now, there is something that you need in order to be able to look at your life so boldly.

It's trust.

Trust that you can endure pain. Trust that you can overcome. Trust that others will be there for you and have your back. Trust that it can get better. Trust in yourself. And I said that I wouldn't give platitudes.

The problem with trust is that it is the antithesis of anxiety. When we're anxious, we try meticulously to prevent as much pain as possible. We don't get into relationships because we don't trust that we can get through a breakup, or we stay in unhealthy relationships because we don't trust that we can live alone. We keep unfulfilling jobs because we don't believe we can do better or we don't want to risk the rejection of losing out on the promotion. Because so much of anxiety is about preventing pain, we often rob ourselves of opportunities where we can witness our resilience. We don't give ourselves a chance to see what happens when we fall in love, when we end an unsatisfying relationship, or when we take a new position.

As a therapist, I see every day what happens when people's worst fears come true. At first, it's usually hell on earth. But then, trust me on this—it's freedom. There's liberation in knowing that you are no longer shackled to your anxiety. It no longer owns you.

Now we're about to go deep with concerning statistics and I know we're only a few pages in. If you think it might be too much, take a breather, skim what's ahead in the next paragraph, and decide whether you're ready for it. Just reading this book is the start of practicing sitting with discomfort and not avoiding your anxiety.

When we're anxious, we so often doubt our own strength. We forget that we can endure. As Glennon Doyle writes in her book *Untamed*, we distrust our ability to #dohardthings. This is why you see such unsettling outcomes in this country. The suicide rate, where we lose 130 people a day,[2] the opioid crisis, where over 10 million Americans over the age of twelve have misused opioids in the past year,[3] and the fact that we have one divorce in this country every forty-two seconds[4] are all examples of our difficulty sitting with pain and trusting that life gets better.

Now, to be clear, every instance of suicide, substance use, and divorce has unique factors warranting their own caveats. However, when we look at these trends collectively, they speak to a larger problem. They highlight our need for avoidance—to run away from pain. Our fears tell us that it's just too difficult and so we flee with wild abandon, hoping that pain will never find us. Sadly, it's often waiting for us at home in other forms—loneliness, disappointment in ourselves, and an even bigger dose of anxiety for whenever the "next time" comes.

So, if you've been stuck on the couch, telling yourself that you're just "not ready," I'm here to help you get your life back. If you have always struggled with facing fears, I'm here to offer you a road map. Your anxiety doesn't need to win any longer. Now, this doesn't mean you won't be uncomfortable. In fact, you will be really freaking uncomfy at a lot of points as you get stronger and put yourself out there again.

And, I would argue, isn't that what you ultimately want, though? To live the life that is meaningful to you? To not let your anxiety call the shots on your future? Personally, I consider it my greatest goal as a clinician to not let anxiety be the reason my clients have regrets or disappointments in their lives.

Let's hit the pause button, though, before we go on. I'd be remiss if I didn't clarify how different anxiety can look for each of us. For some of us, anxiety is a privilege—for others, anxiety is an almost inevitable by-product that emerges as a result of the destructiveness of our society.

For example, anxiety can be a privilege when you're losing sleep at night wondering whether you should go to a school in state or across the country. Or when you're deciding whether to purchase a house or stay in your apartment for another year. What about choosing between a corporate job and pursuing an entrepreneurial journey? Anxiety is a privilege if you can't decide how you want to spend your money—but you have enough of it regardless. All are understandable conditions where anxiety may bubble up, but privilege is inherent, to varying extents, in each example.

Anxiety is *not* a privilege when you worry that a bullet will rip through your house because your neighborhood is frequently hit with gun violence. Anxiety is not a privilege when you have to decide between buying groceries, getting gas, and paying your medical bills. Or when you're scared that Border Patrol could tell you that you need to leave your residence immediately. How about when you're scared that you may be attacked if you wear a pagri or hijab, because you are trans, or because you appear to be of a certain race or ethnicity? In these situations, anxiety is not a privilege—anxiety is often a given and is a justifiable worry for many.

As a cisgender, white, straight, Protestant, socioeconomically stable, housed, well-educated, able-bodied, neurotypical, slim adult woman, I realize that I have had an inordinate amount of privilege in my life thus far. There are so many opportunities that I have had because of my privilege (as well as the privilege that my parents have had, along with the generations before them who were endowed with ample opportunities). Heck, I get to write this book as a psychologist because of the massive amount of privilege that I have had and con- tinue to have. I have been able to afford an education, have a home where I can comfortably write (if sometimes begrudgingly), and eat all the English muffins I can muster that are in plentiful supply in my refrigerator. Indeed, in many ways the anxiety that I have experienced in my life has come from a place of privilege rather than dire need or real danger.

I will never claim to know the experience of anxiety that is all too real for those living with marginalized identities and/or residing in sometimes unsafe communities. I have heard many precious cli- ent stories that reveal how harrowing and heartbreaking it is to walk into a bathroom and not know whether someone will be there waiting to hurt you. To stay behind on a school trip because your citizenship status does not let you travel outside of the country (and, worse yet, to never get to return to your homeland for fear that you will not get to come back to your present country of residence). To feel like you have to hide your identity at Thanksgiving dinner because your family will make fun of you for loving who you love. While I hold tremendous empathy and a sense of humble openness to continue to learn, I will never truly know what these experiences are like. I do know, though, that it breaks my heart if you are reading this and you know this anxiety all too well because you have lived or are continuing to live through these pains.

It never should have been this way. I ache knowing that you ache.

Anxiety looks different for each of us, depending on the storied life that each of us has led. We all have different paths that have brought us here to this page. Even as you read this, you may find that you've been comparing your anxieties to those of others. Perhaps you have been guilting yourself for feeling anxious when others "have it so much worse." You minimize your pain, feeling that it pales in light of what someone else has gone through. Or maybe you have been validating your own experience while belittling another's, saying, "It's not that bad." Perhaps you scoff, saying, "Some people are such babies."

Yet I will say this: **Pain is pain. Anxiety is anxiety.**

No matter the symptom—the physical sensations, the ruminative distress, feeling like a victim in your own body—anxiety is universally and undeniably uncomfortable. It can bring us all to our knees, no matter what set it off. It can have a grip on us that is unshakable. When this happens, our acknowledgment of that pain is sometimes our best course of action. Shaming ourselves that we "shouldn't" feel anxiety often only amplifies distress.

And while these circumstances are often beyond our control, we get to choose how we show up in the aftermath. Whether a situation is self-created or the result of life unexpectedly handing us a juicy peach through the thorns, we get to decide how we respond to our challenges and choose whether to take a bite or not.

Anxiety is the purgatory in between that tells you you're just not ready, though. It tells you that you'll make a fool of yourself. It says that it won't be worth it. It whispers in your ear that people will judge you. While we sit and stare at that disarmingly juicy peach of an opportunity day after day, eventually either that peach rots or another bird comes along and eats it. So much of the time we can let our anxiety sour our future as we tell ourselves that we need "just a little more time."

So I'm here to tell you: eat the damn peach.

Personally, I don't think anxiety should have the authority to determine the outcome of your life. As you'll see in our work together, that means that you may do incredibly meaningful things in your life and anxiety may be there the whole time. What matters is that you make the choices that serve you—not your anxiety.

Part of why I specialize in anxiety and love treating all forms of it is because it's highly treatable. Anxiety is one of the most researched psychological experiences and there are several interventions that have been shown to be effective for various populations. We'll be covering these throughout this book, with a special focus on acceptance and commitment therapy (ACT), developed by Dr. Steven C. Hayes. With the hundreds of clients I've treated, I've seen ACT help time and time again because it's a completely different approach from the traditional response of trying to make anxiety "go away."

ACT is your candid, no-nonsense friend acknowledging that, truthfully, we can't always make anxiety stop. However, we get to decide how we want to live our lives—even if anxiety is here for the ride. We choose whom we date, where we live, what we do—we don't need to wait for anxiety to disappear in order to start taking purposeful action. That's why I see tremendous beauty in this framework: ACT recognizes that life is painful while reminding us that we don't need this pain to be the reason we stop living our lives the way we want.

Part of why I love ACT so much is that I've seen how life-changing it's been not only for my clients but in my own life as well. While it's been a common dogma for therapists to rarely self-disclose, I think it's important to be a real person and share my personal experiences with you. As we say, sharing our own stories when it's for the sake of the client's benefit can be justified. Thus, I hope that in my telling of my own plight with anxiety—and, more importantly, how I've been able to work with it—you will find some relatability and hope.

I want you to know that I empathize with your experience. I'll share more on this later, but I've lived my own lifelong battle with a phobia that evolved into a panic disorder. Since I was a little kid, I've experienced what's called emetophobia—a fear of vomit—both when others get sick and when I myself feel sick. It's not uncommon when I get triggered that I have a full-blown panic attack where I will shake uncontrollably, struggle to speak, and feel nauseous. If you've ever had a panic attack, you know how brutal it can be.

I've been to therapy for these experiences throughout my life and I've seen what has worked . . . and what hasn't. As you'll see throughout this book, talk therapy is just one path to healing. There are so many options, both evidence based and less researched (but heartily client endorsed), that can work for you. I invite you to have an open mind about what you need—and not just blindly follow what someone is telling you to do. Whether it's acupuncture, massage therapy, exercise, art therapy, or naturopathy, there are so many tools that go beyond a Westernized approach to care. While I'm all for well-researched methods, I'm just as much for client advocacy and culturally centered forms of healing. If it *feels* like it is helping you (even though the research may not strictly back it up), then that is enough when it comes to anxiety management.

There's also something I want to be clear on before we proceed. As a feminist therapist, I think it's crucial that we eliminate the power differential where I am perceived as the expert and you, the client, are perceived as the student in need. If anything, you and I are both just trying to figure this thing out together. Yes, I worked hard to get my credentials and my license number as a practicing psychologist. I would hope that the time, dollars, and energy would allow me to proffer something fruitful and valuable to you. But at the end of the day, I'm right alongside you—coming to this work humbly and with a sense of open curiosity.

I'm also sharing composite stories from the therapy space based on recurrent themes that I have seen from some of the hundreds of clients I have worked with, in the hope that you will see your stories in theirs. All client identities and life details have been protected so that their confidentiality is maintained at all times. The demographics and experiences I will share are compilations of different cases, so that no one client is recognizable. Thus, if you were to go out looking for Mikaela, Jacob, Nikita, or any of the "clients" you're soon to meet, you wouldn't find them, as the specific person described in each chapter doesn't in fact exist in the real world. What does exist are the thoughts, feelings, and actions portrayed here in this book as I have seen these patterns of anxiety play out time and time again. As you hear these client journeys, may you be heartened in knowing that you are not alone in your own battle with anxiety and pain. So much is kept behind the closed doors (or the encrypted Zoom room) of a therapy session, and for good reason. There is a sacredness in session. However, here is an opportunity for you to know that you are not alone and to have your concerns normalized as I take you alongside these example client journeys. Perhaps it will give you a different vantage point as you look at your own journey.

I also want to be mindful of where you're at. You may have some ruminative worry that annoys you a bit . . . or you may have a debilitating level of anxiety that makes it nearly impossible to leave your home. Anxiety is on such a wide spectrum, and I want to respect where on that spectrum you are. Go at the pace that works for you throughout this book. While I like to challenge you, I never want you to feel so pushed that it becomes punitive.

Approaching anxiety is always a dance. While avoidance is not the answer, neither is making you feel so overwhelmed that you're flooded and retraumatized. I'm going to invite you to lean into the discomfort as much as you can while respecting your boundaries. Do what you can. As you'll see, each time we get through something a little scary (whether it's reading a bit of text or facing a fear in your lived experience), you'll likely notice that the big waves of fear get a little smaller each time. This is how you build your bandwidth and, ultimately, your anxiety threshold.

If you do find yourself getting panicky or overly activated while reading this book, take a breath. Use a guided mindfulness exercise—the ones from the Calm app are my favorite. Get a cold glass of water and place it on your forehead. This stimulates the vagus nerve, which will help activate your parasympathetic response, slowing down your heart rate and breathing. Get some fresh air if you can. These are ways to ground yourself if at any point you become too overwhelmed. We'll cover more of these vagus nerve regulation strategies in chapter 9, if you'd like to bookmark that section in advance. Remember, we go at your pace. I do like to challenge you so that you see yourself grow, but ultimately you are in charge. Let's dive in.

CHAPTER ONE

FACING YOUR OCEAN

~~~~~~~~~~~~~~~~~~~~~~~~~~~~~~~~

WHY THE WATER AND YOUR MIND AREN'T ALL THAT DIFFERENT

I always like to start my sessions with a nice cup of hot green tea. Sometimes I'll light a candle and I'll open my window to hear the leaves rustling outside. As I settle in each morning, and Mochi, my little Siamese cat, gets into his therapy chair, we review my schedule of clients for the day. I start to mentally prepare myself for the people I'm seeing—each one bringing out something different from me. With some there's laughter, with some long pauses, and some need soothing. When I first started seeing Mikaela, I could tell she needed the latter. Imagine a straight, cisgender, Armenian woman in her midthirties with a kind smile and big, green, hopeful eyes. In our early sessions, her tears were spilling out faster than her words. She shared with me that she was at her wit's end. She had near daily panic attacks, woke up vomiting most mornings, and struggled to leave her house because of her fears surrounding the pandemic (which had only intensified after a long-standing history of health anxiety). Her weariness was undeniable to both of us.

Her anxiety was having tangible effects on her life. She avoided going to the doctor because she was afraid of the potential procedures they might do, like drawing blood (which was particularly triggering, given her needle phobia). Sex was painful for her, and she experienced what is called genito-pelvic pain/penetration disorder, where it was difficult or nearly impossible for her to enjoy having sex with her boyfriend. She had become incredibly self-conscious about being intimate with him and began to experience anticipatory anxiety for their future encounters. Problematically, he would shame her about this. This only intensified her anxiety around sex even more. Not to mention she felt isolated and overwhelmed as she prepared to finish graduate school and get ready for her next steps. With all this stress, she would nap for long periods of time and hide out in her apartment. She felt like sleep was the only escape from the mental prison of her mind.

Mikaela's story is sadly not unique. Even as you read it, you may be identifying with different elements and believing this story was written about you. While the content may vary, you will likely empathize with the feelings shared in each client's experience.

That's the thing—anxiety is a tie that binds us all. We all have different roots and reasons for it, but our bodies make it known nevertheless. And if you're unprepared for it, it can feel like your body is betraying you in the worst way.

Mikaela had not yet identified the links between her lived experiences, her physical sensations, and her anxiety. In turn she was absolutely bewildered by her body. You may have wondered this yourself—befuddled as to why you're nauseous each morning, why you choke when you swallow, or why you're getting constipated or having diarrhea on a weekly (or daily) basis. You may have sought medical doctors, looking for plausible answers and getting what feels like an insufficient response: "It's probably *just* anxiety." As if it's that innocuous.

I've felt confused and trapped by my own body at times. It started in high school when I struggled to eat because of frequent nausea and stomach pain. I lost fifteen pounds within two months. I was told there was "no clear diagnosis," even after I was given an ultrasound and CT scan. That's right—I wasn't even told it was anxiety that I was grappling with, and, looking back, I remember never being asked about any symptoms of anxiety. It continued in college when I literally peed my pants from a bladder that couldn't hold itself (for the sake of this story I wish I could tell you I was intoxicated but I was all too sober). I went on to have several urine tests and, again, no clear answers and not one mention of anxiety. I've since learned that frequent urination is actually a fairly common sign of anxiety.[5]

When you don't know what anxiety looks like, the signals that your body is sending can be even more alarming. Incidentally, this often only worsens the anxiety, and the physical and mental symptoms continue to amplify. It can feel like we're in completely unknown waters and we can't see the bottom. You may know that feeling if you've ever been diving or snorkeling and you can't see the floor of the ocean and start to panic. There's an actual name for this phobia: thalassophobia, where we fear the vastness and emptiness of the ocean. I know some of you are adding this to your list of symptoms as we speak.

I think it's actually quite helpful to utilize the water as a metaphor for our distress, and you'll see me build on this visualization throughout the book. Whether or not we have a phobia of the ocean, there are several parallels between our minds and the sea. Let me explain how the ocean and our minds are quite similar:

1. **The great unknown:** We've only explored about 20 percent of the ocean in its entirety.[6] In fact, a greater percentage of the surface of the moon and the planet Mars have been mapped out compared to our ocean floor.[7] Similarly, we continue to identify and understand new areas within the brain. Researchers are differentiating more complexities within our neocortex on a regular basis, having named 180 separate areas in our cerebral cortex.[8] We are evolving to better understand how our genetics interact with our environment to create our lived experiences

and physical symptoms, but the unique intersectionality in the brain continues to remain largely unexplained.

2. **The unpredictability:** Yes, we can draw out the expected pattern of the tides, but if you've ever been in the ocean, you know the sudden power of a wave knocking against your back. It can take our breath away and topple us over with a sudden smack. We fear the same unpredictability in our own lives. Worse yet, we doubt our ability to endure, making us feel like we are one phone call away from dissolution.

3. **The sharks in our waters:** There are so many harmful experiences, harmful people, and systemic injustices that make our lives feel unsafe. Just as we would feel if we were to see a shark fin pop out of the water five feet away from us, we have an instantaneous physiological response when we feel physically and emotionally threatened each day in our communities. We'll dive into this more in depth in chapter 6 as we look at the specific types of sharks in our waters.

Whether you've never been in the ocean or you've swum in the water every day, we all can resonate with the power and unpredictability of the ocean, similar to how we may currently be relating to our anxiety. I have seen time and time again how these kinds of metaphors can ground the sometimes intangible concepts and frame them in a whole new way that is easier to wrap our minds around.

THE CHOICE TO SWIM OR SINK WHEN ANXIETY HITS

By the time I saw Mikaela, she had been swimming in some rough waters for a long time. Her body was tapped out, exhausted from being surrounded by metaphorical shark-infested waters for years. Indeed, Mikaela's long-standing battle with anxiety had led to an add-on of depression, making her feel hopeless that her situation would improve. This is not uncommon, as a worldwide survey found that 45.7 percent of those experiencing depression also had a history of one or more anxiety disorders during their lifetimes.[9] Perhaps you can relate, feeling depleted by what feels like an endless monotony of panic to start your morning, exhaustion throughout your day, and dread as night approaches.

That's why I've wanted to write this book. I've seen too many people inundated by the anxiety (and subsequent depression) and they've reached a state of hopelessness. As someone who was having multiple panic attacks a week, unable to go out to restaurants, and dreading getting on planes, I've been there myself. A major part of why I wanted to write this book was to give you a sense of hope that it can get better. I've seen it with client after client and I know you can have a similar story with a happier-ever-after.

It's not always going to be easy. You're going to have to do the work. Sometimes it's going to be uncomfortable as you ride through the waves of anxiety and see what's on the other side. But I can promise you that this book can start to give you your power—not your control—back. That wording is intentional.

Anxiety makes us *crave* control. If only we could have the security and predictability we seek, then we would have permission to be at peace. As you'll see throughout this book, there is no such thing as ultimate security and predictability. When we come to face the reality of how little control we often have in our lives (something most of us had to see collectively during the pandemic), there can actually be liberation rather than debilitation. I know this is counterintuitive. But it's in acknowledging our situation and choosing our intentional response to this lack of control that we get our power back. When it feels like life is happening to us, our response and how we handle our situation is our fortitude. This is what can ground us. No one can ever take that away no matter how uncontrollable a situation may be.

Let me put this concept into context. As I mentioned earlier, my client Mikaela had avoided going to the doctor for years because of the uncontrollable reaction her body would have when she was in any medical setting. Like many clients, she would cry, shake, and sometimes even pass out because of the anxiety coursing through her veins. Her response was to prevent herself from getting medical care because of the powerful grip that her anxiety held her in. This came to a head when she wanted to get the COVID vaccine but felt paralyzed by the thought of getting injected by a needle.

Part of Mikaela's getting her power back included learning about how the fear manifested for her. She took steps—by both identifying the thoughts she was believing, and integrating medical interventions such as taking prescriptions from a psychiatrist—so that she would feel physically calmer throughout the process. She asked for support, bringing her sister with her so that she didn't have to endure the stress alone. By taking these actions, Mikaela was ultimately able to get vaccinated, and it got a little easier for her each time. This was her taking ownership of the situation, even when the anxiety felt out of control.

We can do this collectively as a society as well. When the uncontrollable happens, we do not have to sit idly by. When the Supreme Court rules that women do not have a say over their bodies, we can march. When an eighteen-year-old can buy assault rifles without any form of a background check, we can call and write our senators to demand change. When we watch home after home burn down or flood out because of our climate crisis, we can call for greater protection of our planet and reduce our impact individually by changing our modes of transportation and cutting back on our use of nonessential material goods. This is the collective power that can ground us when it feels like the world is literally drowning us in despair.

Anxiety makes us want to run away, telling us that it's "all too much." And yes, it is too much. It's not uncommon that each week we find ourselves crying at our TVs, shaking our heads at the latest news alerts, and feeling immobilized when the same tragedies happen over and over again. But that's how anxiety wins. That's how the uncontrollable feels even more out of control. That's when we start to feel like we're drowning in the waters around us and not learning how to swim through.

THE MOST IMPORTANT FIRST STEP WE CAN TAKE

I want to emphasize: if we're going to turn the tide on our anxiety, it starts by getting our power back. It's when we choose how to respond in a meaningful way with action rather than apathy that anxiety dwindles. And what's one of the most important choices we can make when it comes to working through anxiety?

Educating ourselves.

Part of why anxiety feels so scary is because we don't understand it. We feel that we're at the mercy of our minds and our bodies. And yet there's a powerful phrase coined by the psychiatrist Dan Siegel, "Name it to tame it."[10] If we can understand the thoughts, feelings, and physical sensations that can come on suddenly or those that last for months on end, we can begin to feel like we have a grasp on our situation. It doesn't necessarily mean that we can control or make these symptoms go away, but by understanding the underpinnings of our distress, we can often deflate our sense of alarm.

So let's learn together. We'll be covering in the next chapter why exactly we're more anxious than ever from a sociological standpoint. Before we do that, though, it's imperative that we break down the biology behind anxiety. So many of us blame ourselves for our distress when, in actuality, we're not giving our brains and our bodies their due credit for going into uncontrollable hyperdrive. Instead, we often panic further because we're so confused by why our minds and our physical beings are acting out.

Much of our anxiety stems from a little almond-size region housed deep inside the brain called the amygdala. As powerful as it is, it takes up only about 0.3 percent of the volume of the brain.[11] The amygdala operates under a delicate balance. If it is overly sensitive, it's not uncommon that you'll see folks experience heightened awareness, avoidance, and a general sense of distrust toward others. If it's underactive, you'll see people engage in more risk-taking behaviors, as was mentioned in the introduction in the case of Alex Honnold's free climb in Yosemite. Interestingly, agitation and anger have also been tied to the amygdala, which may explain why irritability can be a common symptom of an anxious presentation.[12]

No matter what your amygdala looks like, anxiety can take a different shape in each of our brains. Where we experience activation—or a lack of activation—in our brains can make a difference. Studies looked at how there may be different subsets under the anxiety umbrella, including how these symptoms present themselves neurologically.[13] For example, some of us may be chronic worriers, ruminating about our past experiences and fretting about our futures. We tend to see this more with generalized anxiety, OCD, or social anxiety, for example. Others experience distinct episodes of panic, noticing things such as a racing heart, difficulty breathing, or sweating when they're placed in a situation that pushes their specific trigger buttons. These folks may function with less day-to-day worrying, but if you place them in settings where they're afraid (think of Michaela with her needle phobia), it can lead to a level-ten panic attack with an activated fight-or-flight response. Thus, diagnoses such as phobias or panic disorder tend to fit the bill here. Some of us luck out and experience both subsets of anxiety. What's fascinating about the findings from the research is that those who have a general sense of worry showed more left-brain activity whereas those who were more panicky with hyperarousal showed more right-brain activity.[14] What does this mean?

It means that anxiety is not a one-size-fits-all. Yes, we can resonate generally with what it means to feel anxious, but how we experience it may be entirely different from one person to the next. Knowing how your anxiety manifests for you is what matters the most. What's going to be most helpful for you may vary greatly depending on what your symptoms look like. For example, if you tend to be a ruminative worrier, practicing mindfulness, though potentially helpful, may actually exacerbate your symptoms as you marinate in your already-well-aware worries. Conversely, if you're a frequent flyer on the panic plane, learning about how to challenge your thoughts (though that is still useful) may not be as effective as learning grounding strategies and doing body work to soothe a nervous system that's on red alert.

This is potentially why you may have been getting so frustrated with yourself. You may have been using the wrong interventions to treat your form of anxiety. That's why it's so important to understand how anxiety paints itself in your life. Don't compare your picture to someone else's. We may use the same paint, but each canvas can look very different.

A NEW WAVE TO RIDE:
Which form of anxiety do you tend to notice more for yourself? Or would you say that you experience both? Take some time to reflect on how your anxiety shows up, physically and emotionally.

Mikaela learned through our work that she had a blend of both types of anxiety. She would worry about a panoply of things (some real, some imagined) while also having specific activators that would send her body into a ricochet of tears, trembling, and trouble speaking. What we found is that while adding supplementation with vitamins and minerals made a beneficial difference in her symptoms, it wasn't enough when she would get triggered by the thought of having to go to the doctor for an annual exam, for example (something that she had put off well into her thirties). She was also finding that some of her physical symptoms were holding on tightly, especially her nausea and frequent vomiting in the morning.

Though not formerly diagnosed, I'd hypothesize that Mikaela was suffering from something called cyclic vomiting disorder (CVD), where a person tends to get sick around the same time just about every day. While the Mayo Clinic cites that there is "no apparent cause" for why people experience CVD, I have to wonder whether the culprit may in fact be anxiety much of the time.[15] And while this nausea can hit at any time of day, it's not uncommon that clients see this queasiness first thing in the morning.

This may be related to what's called the cortisol awakening response, as our cortisol levels are highest in the first hour after waking up.[16] Given that cortisol is considered the stress hormone, released by the adrenal glands when we feel fear or are overwhelmed, this makes sense. Once you add caffeine to your morning routine (which can also give the jitters), low blood sugar from not eating a balanced breakfast, and perhaps a hangover from trying to drink your fears away the night prior, you have a recipe for the morning sickies. Mikaela was batting for three, as she would regularly down two cups of coffee, eat sugary cereal for breakfast, and nurse a hangover from drinking a few beers the night before. Before long, she was unfortunately kneeling by the porcelain, feeling more discouraged and frustrated than ever. As the cycle continued, she began experiencing anticipatory anxiety as the final cherry on this unwanted sundae. She worried that it would happen again, only amplifying her initial distress.

When physical symptoms are taking over, such as vomiting, frequent crying, insomnia, and exhaustion, as was the case with Mikaela, it's important to look at the whole tool kit of resources. This is when medication can make a big difference. While she was very hesitant to do so at first, Mikaela began considering the possibility of seeing a psychiatrist, as she was at her wit's end with her body's antics.

After carefully deliberating, Mikaela decided that she would give medication a try if a psychiatrist thought it would be useful. I helped her find a provider whom she felt comfortable with (PsychologyToday.com is a great place to find both therapists and psychiatrists who take your insurance). After her initial appointment, Michaela's doctor prescribed her an SSRI, or a selective serotonin reuptake inhibitor, which is an antidepressant that typically takes about four to six weeks to go into effect. Mikaela soon noticed that her morning nausea all but disappeared, her uncontrollable crying lessened, and her panic attacks were greatly reduced. She told me that, for her, taking medication was a game changer. I saw the difference, too. She started laughing in her sessions, she cut back on her drinking because she didn't need it as much to cope, and, heck, she even got a puppy. Ultimately she told me before we ended our work together: "I'm so glad that I gave the medication a chance to help me."

Now, of course, the decision to take medication is highly personal. While some people have said that medication has turned them into a "zombie" or changed their personality, it may be worth finding out why they felt that way before we jump to similar conclusions (for example, perhaps it wasn't the right dosage or prescription for that specific person). It's not for everyone, but I also know that I've seen many skeptical clients experience how medication indeed changes their personalities for the better—where they actually feel like themselves again, the people they were before the anxiety took hold of their lives. Maybe you owe it to yourself to see whether this could be of value to you if you're feeling fed up. Besides, if you're already self-medicating with alcohol, cannabis, or other substances anyway (and feeling dependent on them), perhaps that's an indicator that another source of support, such as prescription medication, could be helpful.

There's no need to judge yourself (or others) if you need medication to support you. There's nothing "wrong" with you. We can all have imbalances in our bodies and brains, and it's an act of self-care to give our bodies what they need. Just as we wouldn't judge someone for taking a probiotic if they wanted to improve their gut flora or a supplement if they had a vitamin D deficiency, we needn't judge someone for wanting to have more balance in their brain by taking a prescribed medication. We can't always control an overactive amygdala or a brain that doesn't want to dance with the serotonin or norepinephrine (two neurotransmitters and hormones that can play a key part in anxiety and depression) floating around in our heads. That's not our fault, just like it's not our fault if we don't have perfect vision, scoliosis (yours truly), or a torn ACL. Sometimes it just happens, and we can do something about it.

That being said, you may be reading this and see medication as a last resort given your cultural, historical, and/or personal background. That's perfectly alright, too. While some diagnoses require more of a pharmacological intervention like schizophrenia or bipolar disorder, anxiety can often abate with several other tools and coping skills that don't rely on medication to be effective.

We get to decide how we respond. We can choose to help ourselves by accepting our reality. Sometimes, that means taking medication, supplements, or probiotics, or changing our diet so that we can give our brains and bodies the best chance to feel better. Other times, it's exercising more regularly, working on our mindset, and engaging more social supports. There is no one-size-fits-all model.

If you have no idea where to start, call your insurance company and ask for a list of providers near you. You can also call 211 for essential community services in your area (available throughout the United States as well as Puerto Rico). I also mentioned PsychologyToday.com as my favorite online platform to find therapists, psychiatrists, support groups, and inpatient treatment programs. For clients looking for more diverse therapy experiences, Therapy for Black Girls, Therapy for Black Men, Therapy for Latinx, and Asian Mental Health Collective are also great resources. If you attend a university or college (and even if you don't), call their student counseling center for a list of referrals—they will have a set of names on hand for you. Another pro tip: nearly all clinical psychology graduate programs for doctoral students offer community clinics in their surrounding area for an incredibly affordable rate. We would see clients for as low as five dollars, depending on what clients could afford. Granted, you are working with student therapists, but they are working closely under a licensed supervisor. This can be a great budget option.

WE ARE MORE THAN OUR BODIES, THOUGH

Treating our bodies' symptoms is rarely enough, though. In the same way that our bodies impact our brain health and our brains' neurochemistry impacts our overall physical health, our environment, relationships, and experiences impact our mental health as well. Known as the biopsychosocial model, which was developed by the late George Engel in 1977, this framework is still relevant today as we consider how our current societal stressors, our personal histories, and our intersectional identities interact with our DNA and brain chemistry to make up our collective well-being.[17,18]

This held true for Mikaela as well. When we considered her family history and relational dynamics, her current stressors started making even more sense. We learned that her father was quite anxious himself, though he never sought treatment for his distress. Instead, he would indoctrinate Mikaela with "recommendations" that were meant to protect her but only heightened her anxiety more. This was often veiled as fatherly love, as he was "looking out for her." What Mikaela walked away with was learning to assume the worst so that she wouldn't be disappointed. She came to expect that others would dislike her, so she would be exceedingly agreeable (a common trope that many women are taught), and she overworked herself to keep others happy. Needless to say, Mikaela soon became a hamster on the people-pleaser wheel and she couldn't keep up.

When Mikaela entered into her most recent relationship, she carried with her all of these familial "words of wisdom." Her people-pleasing, agreeableness, and fear of disappointing others were in full force, especially in the bedroom. It's vulnerable enough to have sex with a partner—and that's when things are good. With her boyfriend, her distress only intensified as she would find her body uncontrollably blocking his entry. To her increasing embarrassment, he was *not happy* when he was denied access to her body through no fault of her own. Because of a lifetime of blaming herself, Mikaela became frustrated with herself and she felt it was "understandable" that her boyfriend would be mad at her when they were unable to have sex. She wondered, "What's wrong with me?"

Mikaela's anxiety was confusing her so much that she didn't know what was up and what was down. I see this happen frequently, as our anxiety makes us doubt ourselves and question our ability to know what's okay and what isn't. Sometimes a helpful question to ask ourselves is "If this were happening to a friend, would I be okay with it?" And if we follow up with "Well, no . . . but it's different because it's happening to me," this is our cue to take a closer look at why we apply different rules to ourselves.

As we talked this through in session, I saw the color drain from Mikaela's cheeks. As she considered another vantage point, she realized that if a friend told her about a partner shaming them for not being able (or simply not wanting) to have sex, she would not be okay with it. In fact, she said she would consider it assault. When she realized this, she felt sick to her stomach. She was seething with anger that this had happened to her. While she was mad at him for doing that to her, she was also mad at herself for allowing it to happen . . . many times over. I made it clear to Mikaela that she did nothing wrong. She shouldn't have ever been put in that situation. It was not okay what happened to her, and her boyfriend's behavior was inexcusable.

Though Mikaela is not a real person, her story is all too common. Sadly, I've seen this story play out with too many women, and some men, in my practice.

Mikaela saw more clearly after that session. The shroud of anxiety had been lifted and she realized just how unacceptable her boyfriend's behavior was, and that it was a likely indicator of additional forms of abuse in the future. Within a week or so, she ended it. (Are you clapping a little bit internally?)

It was a proud therapy mama moment as I watched Mikaela take that step for herself. As therapists, we want you to be empowered in the choices that you make in your life. What you decide to do is solely up to you. That being said, there are certain situations, like when abuse is present, that we will take a more directive approach and inform you of our concern for your physical safety. This was one of those times, and I was glad to see Mikaela get out of harm's way.

As time went on, Mikaela and I continued to process the relationship with her *ex*-boyfriend. She came to see that his behavior was in fact abusive and she adamantly noted that she would never accept that behavior again. She took some time on her own to heal her relationship with her body. She began doing Pilates, went to physical therapy (yes, they have that for genito-pelvic pain disorder), and started exploring masturbation to build more comfortability with her body. And when she was ready, she started to date again. She knew which red flags to look out for and was no longer excessively accommodating. She learned how to be alert to any potential signs of disrespect and only continued with partners who were patient and made her feel comfortable and safe. She did the work and it paid off.

LEARNING TO RIDE RATHER THAN RESIST YOUR WAVES

Ultimately, Mikaela learned how to ride the waves of her anxiety, rather than resist them. If we can come to accept, like Mikaela did, that life will provide innumerable waves, we can start to see that every wave that comes eventually goes. It doesn't mean it's easy. It can hurt like heck. And yes, we'll cover what to do when a wave absolutely knocks you on your ass. But with many of them, we *can* ride them out. We often just don't give ourselves the credit that we can get through it.

We often scare ourselves silly with the "what-ifs." We fret over getting in a car crash, having food poisoning, or someone making fun of us. And this worrying is not necessarily maladaptive when used appropriately. Our brains have evolved to do this as a form of protection.[19] Worrying helps us put on a seat belt and not text and drive so that we don't get in a car crash. It reminds us to wash our hands when we're cooking with raw chicken. It helps us to make sure we don't have spinach in our teeth before we go to a party (I wish I worried more about this one).

But here's the thing: so many feared "what-ifs" never actually come to pass. In fact, the clinical psychologist Melanie Greenberg writes in her book, *The Stress-Proof Brain*, that about "85% of the things people worry about never happen."[20] If we reminded ourselves of this and began trusting ourselves to face the situations we find ourselves in, we may actually enjoy the experience a little bit more.

Instead of tensing up, looking over our shoulders for each potential setback, we can start settling in and surfing the waves as they come. Some we'll ride out better than others. We may fall off the board spectacularly, but we can laugh at ourselves and learn from it, instead of shaming ourselves for looking like a fool. This is where you can choose to approach yourself with kindness when you stumble.

At the end of the day, we're all doing the best that we can. Giving ourselves some grace as we navigate each wave (because each one is different) may be just the ticket. If there's something that you start to simmer on as you go through this book, I hope it's a deep, heartfelt sense of knowing that it's okay to be tender with yourself. Your anxiety may have told you for years that you need to be strict, uncompromising, and callous with yourself. It may have told you that without that brutal upholding of yourself, you will fall apart.

I'm here to tell you that it doesn't have to be that way. If you're willing to lean back and embrace your inner self, I know that you'll come to see that life is a heck of a lot easier when you float along with the highs and lows than when you grit your teeth and bear down for any tiny bump coming up. I got you. More important: you've got *you*.

CHAPTER TWO

WHEN THE WATERS OF ANXIETY ARE ALL AROUND YOU

When Nikita came onto my Zoom screen I could barely see her eyes because her head hung so low. She was scared to start therapy, as she'd never done it before and all she had to base it on was what she'd seen in TV shows and movies. Identifying at the time as a Black, Christian, straight, cisgender woman, she was trembling as she was so afraid to tell me what was bothering her. I shared with her that my goal as a therapist was to create a totally nonjudgmental space, and that there was nothing she could say that could shock me. Hearing this, she started to open up; as she would later tell me, she'd never before had a safe space to fully explore who she was.

She disclosed that for years she had been battling addictions to vaping, getting drunk, and then online shopping. After she'd grapple with each long day, this cycle would be Nikita's way of numbing out from the world so that she didn't have to sit with the full weight of the pain. Over time, this led to her feeling disempowered, as she lost faith in her ability to feel in control of her life. With thousands of dollars in debt from vape cartridges, liquor, and shopping sprees, she no longer trusted herself. She felt like she was a victim of her own mind and body, and seriously doubted that she could change the cycle of addictive behaviors that were taking up her evenings and ruining her mornings.

You likely know how this feels if you've experienced any kind of addiction: you steel yourself at the start of the day, promising yourself that this time it will be different, only to be disappointed when the same patterns occur that night. You go to bed feeling ashamed, yet you promise yourself that tomorrow you'll make a change. This is how the cycle felt for Nikita—day in, day out.

Nikita, like many of us, felt the weight of the world on her shoulders. Struggling to get a job that inspired her yet still paid the bills, feeling judged by her family for not being more "successful," and trying to better understand herself in a haze of anxiety were all a part of her daily concerns. Not to mention, her brain was jarred by the constant news cycle that made her feel afraid to drive in her car, walk home to her apartment, or go out on a date. Basically, it felt daunting just to be alive, she'd tell me.

If you can relate to Nikita's never-ending list of fears (and if you've got some of your own special flavor), you can come sit with us.

Just as we are watching our planet's destruction through global warming, we are watching Millennials, just like Nikita, and Generation Z grapple with anxiety like never before. I wouldn't be surprised to see Generation Alpha (born between 2010 and 2024) follow in our footsteps, given that a significant event in their childhood was the COVID-19 crisis.

Unfortunately, the waters we've been in have always been murky. Every generation has their landmark, defining events, and rather than experiencing collective healing, where we can reconnect to a sense of hope, we have been experiencing generational trauma, which can lead us to lose faith in humanity and our personal role in it.

To better understand the pain we're experiencing now, we need to identify what brought us here in the first place. In a fascinating survey done by Visual Capitalist, the Generational Power Index (GPI), the Silent Generation (born between 1928 and 1945), Baby Boomers (born between 1946 and 1964), Generation X (born between 1965 and 1980), and Millennials (born between 1981 and 1996) were asked what they thought were the top ten defining historical moments during their lifetimes. I'll share that data with you in a moment.

Before I go on, though, I think it may be helpful for you to reflect on what you believe to be the most defining historical moments for your generation. I did this exercise with Nikita as well. Given that she kept blaming herself that she wasn't "resilient enough" to manage her anxiety, I thought it was important to help put her anxiety in context. The reality is, when we consider all the pain that has happened in recent years, and in the hundreds of years prior that have led up to this point, it makes a lot more sense why we're more stressed and scared than ever. It's not that we're not strong enough—it's that there's just been *far too much* that has transpired. We're drowning in it. Nikita certainly was—the drinking, vaping, and online shopping were all ways that she simply tried to distract herself and numb out the pain.

If you keep blaming yourself for not being strong enough like Nikita did, perhaps it's time to consider how all the events that have happened throughout your life could be impacting you. We often don't even realize how much the daily devastation we either witness or hear about correlates with our mental health. So, let's connect the dots. When you look back on your life thus far, what headlines in the news or transformative changes have been significant, culture-shaping moments or tide-turners? Keep in mind, some of these may be positive experiences—it doesn't have to be all bad. In addition, take some time to note your personal top ten defining moments in your own life—including the good and the bad. Noting the monumental moments of our lives, as well as our generation's, can give us helpful data to better understand why we may feel the way that we do (and in turn, why we may be so anxious).

WHAT WOULD YOU SAY ARE THE TOP TEN DEFINING MOMENTS OR MOVEMENTS FOR YOUR GENERATION?

1. _____
2. _____
3. _____
4. _____
5. _____
6. _____
7. _____
8. _____
9. _____
10. _____

WHAT WOULD YOU SAY HAVE BEEN THE TOP TEN DEFINING MOMENTS OR MILESTONES IN YOUR PERSONAL LIFE?

1. _____
2. _____
3. _____
4. _____
5. _____
6. _____
7. _____
8. _____
9. _____
10. _____

As you look at this list, do you see any common themes? Do you see any pivotal moments or markers that may have shaped your perspective? Ask yourself how these key experiences impact you today. Perhaps they led to a sudden change where you immediately saw the world through a different lens, or maybe it was more of a gradual shift where you didn't even notice the changes while they were happening. Pulling our history together, both personal and collective, is pivotal as we narrate our journeys—especially when it comes to our relationship with anxiety. When we're feeling like we can barely see straight because of our stress, it helps to understand how that stress got there in the first place.

Let's now compare your list to what the GPI found. It should also be noted that the #MeToo movement, COVID-19 crisis, and George Floyd's and Breonna Taylor's murders (among too many more) came after this survey was completed, but I'd say it's likely that these significant experiences, among others, would now make the list for many.

Interestingly, when each generation was asked to name the top ten historical events or movements that occurred in their lifetimes that they believed had the greatest impact, they unanimously named September 11, 2001. After that, the answers varied, with the Silent Generation going on to name World War II and JFK's assassination, the latter named by the Baby Boomers as the second-most-impactful event. Gen X and Millennials thought the second-most-impactful historical event was Barack Obama's election.

Millennials also noted the following as meaningful events in this order: the Iraq/Afghanistan wars, the legalization of gay marriage, the tech revolution, the Orlando nightclub shooting, Hurricane Katrina, the Columbine shooting, the death of Osama bin Laden, and the Sandy Hook shooting.[21]

According to an American Psychological Association Stress in America survey,[22] when Gen Z was asked about what they considered significant for their generation, mass shootings topped the list. In fact, 75 percent of those surveyed noted that gun violence was a significant stressor in their lives. Fifty-seven percent of them also endorsed stress about the separation and deportation of immigrant families, something that had not previously made the list in the GPI.

I don't know about you, but when I look at these lists, it seems pretty understandable why we're more anxious than ever. While there are some positive events on that list, such as seeing Barack Obama become the first Black president to take office, and watching our LGBTQIA+ friends get married, there have also been some tremendous losses. Whether we're watching a man take his last breath after eight whole minutes under the knee of a police officer, or hearing about twenty kids and six staff members killed on what should have been a normal December day in Newtown, Connecticut, our souls can feel debilitatingly crushed. It's nearly paralyzing.

Certainly when Nikita, as a self-identified Black woman, went through the list of defining historical events in her life, it became even more explicitly clear how the violence against Black people, daily mass shootings, and the pandemic were all adding to a crushing anxiety for her and making it that much harder for her to feel comfortable leaving her home. Rather than continue to knock herself down for not "coping" better, she slowly began to name how these systemic problems were outside of her immediate control when she zoomed out. After realizing that these near-daily monumental events were undeniably impacting her well-being (and how could they not?), she started to give herself permission to no longer self-blame when it came to the origins of her anxieties. Instead, she acknowledged that she had been doing her best to get through these daily hurdles, and on most days, that was more than enough. For the first time, she could see her own strength reflected back to her. Once she named this, there was no going back.

What happens for you when you look at your own narrative? Are you shaming yourself for not being stronger, even despite what you've gone through? When I look at these findings about these generational events, I can't help but notice there's a common thread that underlies why we are more anxious than ever before. What is it? Without a shift in perspective . . .

We feel utterly powerless.

We feel out of control.

We feel like change will never come.

It's hard to feel hopeful in your country when guns have become the leading cause of childhood morbidity in 2020 and many of your representatives basically refuse to make changes in legislation because their votes are protected by gun lobbyists.[23] It's maddening when they say gun violence is a "mental health issue" but are unwilling to remove the means that allow this violence to happen.

It's hard to trust that things can get better when you wake up, and on the news once again is video footage of a police officer shooting a Black man in the back or while he's sitting in his car. Or you hear of a Chinese grandmother brutally attacked while she's waiting to cross the street because someone believes it's "her fault" that the COVID-19 crisis happened. Another day, another face, another name for us to now say—instead of a person to know—because they're gone.

You start to doubt that things will be different when you have to evacuate your home for the third time this year because there's a fire (in December). Maybe this time you won't get so lucky and you'll drive up to a house shredded to ashes. And yet you hear people denying that climate change is real, and there is a refusal to enact policy that could help protect the planet.

It's scary to be in your body when you learn that what you can do with it won't be fully in your hands anymore when nine people can decide that they no longer believe that you should be allowed this right, even after fifty years of upheld precedent. And then you worry that more of your rights will be taken away.

It's tough to have hope when you're financially worse off compared to your parents and you're barely able to afford rent and you have a job you hate that barely pays off your student loans. In fact, Millennials are considered the first generation that is not exceeding their parents' income and job status.[24] Unable to afford a house and yet pressured to get a college education, we're left with a sense of dread, thinking, "This isn't what I signed up for."

I could go on with this list, but I think you get the gist. No matter how loud we try to make ourselves, our cries seem to fall on deaf ears and, perhaps more important, empty pens.

We're tired. We're doubtful that any of it can make a difference. The wear and tear of anxiety over the years has built up an emotional tartar that has left us calloused. Our skepticism has left us siloed in our social media channels and Netflix caves. Even though we're all collectively hurting, we can feel like no one understands our pain. That was where Nikita was when she came out of her tunnel to tell me her story. She felt like no one would understand her strife, including me, someone who looked very different from her.

HOW WE CAN COME TOGETHER WHEN WE FEEL SO ALONE

Though I have never walked in Nikita's shoes, I wanted to walk alongside her. It took time for us to build trust. It was never an expectation or an obligation for Nikita to share. I wanted her to know that whether it was me or someone else, she got to decide whom she opened up to. It was her story to tell and no one but she was endowed the rights to it.

As we shared space together week after week, we started to create community across the screen. Though perhaps considered taboo by the therapy doctrine of old, I shared parts of my identity with Nikita. Normally, we're instructed to not tell our clients anything about ourselves. You may have experienced this when you asked a simple question to your therapist about their identity and they respond coyly with "What makes you want to know?"

So many clients have shared that it feels hard to open up to someone they know nothing about and Nikita was no exception. She wanted to know who was taking in her narrative before she freely gave it out.

I let Nikita know that I myself identified as a Christian. We talked about what our faith meant to us and how we experienced our religious identification. While we shared this belief framework, we also explored the possible variations in our ideologies and how there may be room for interpretation with our lived faith, especially when it comes to whom we love (more on that in a moment). As Nikita got to know more of me, she allowed me to know more of her. It was in allowing herself to be seen for who she was that she started to give herself permission to see herself fully for the first time.

I saw through our work together that healing is not one-directional. It goes both ways. Just as I had hoped to help Nikita by inviting her into the space fully, embracing all the parts of her identity that she struggled with, she also taught me the power of community. We shared a heart-to-heart connection, rather than a purely psychoeducational experience (as talk therapy can be at times). We saw how coming together, just as two people who were once strangers, was such a salve to the personal and generational pain that we'd both experienced in unique ways.

On the surface, we were two very different women. We looked different and we had very different lived experiences. And yet, as we opened our hearts to each other, making space for the tears, for the silence, and for the confusion that comes with not having all the answers, we started to truly see each other. And with that seeing came a sense of closeness that I believe brought a profound peace for both of us. It didn't diminish the loudness and the pain of the outside world—if anything it gave us more bandwidth to sit with it. As we had been holding our breath before, therapy became a space where the exhale was possible.

I invite you to start seeing other people as well—people who are totally different from you, people whom you would pass by on the street or sit next to on a plane and not give a second thought to. We're all in our own little bubbles, looking down into our phones rather than seeing each other's faces—the faces right in front of us. Yes, we're all wildly different from one another and no one is going to get exactly what you've gone though. We can feel alone pretty quickly by telling ourselves that "no one understands." And sure, no one has had your lived experience. But we do have one thing in common: we are all living together, in this world, *right now*. We're all trying to grapple with the new realities that each day brings. We don't have to go at it alone.

Our ability to empathize can vary, but I do believe that most people want to be there for the people around them. Rather than telling yourself that no one cares about you or that people will only hurt you (indeed, some will), I challenge you to hold on to a hope that there are people—people you don't even know yet—who want to do right by you. There are people who do want to understand. People exist who care that you are hurting. They want to be there for you, in whatever way they can. And perhaps you can be there for someone else as well. We don't have to know all the answers or say all the "right" things to show love for our fellow human beings. Sometimes, we just need to show up and to listen. Your presence alone can be your power to heal yourself and to help offer healing to someone else.

A NEW WAVE TO RIDE:
What are some ways that you can get more connected to your community and the people around you? What stops you from reaching out and how can you break through this fear?

A NEW NARRATIVE IN OUR STORIES

When we learned how to sit together in the space, something powerful happened for Nikita. Knowing that she alone could be a part of a positive change, she was no longer trapped in an endless, hopeless cycle. She felt empowered to take her power back when she saw that she was enough. She no longer just watched the news—she became a part of the news by showing how her voice could make a difference. She began tutoring kids in her neighborhood, she reached out to mentors to better understand her career path, and she protested for causes that she cared about. I saw her anxiety abate as she took bold steps toward her future. She was no longer waiting for someone else's permission.

You can get your power back, too. Yes, our generation may seem defined by our anxiety, but that doesn't have to be how our history is ultimately written. We can take the pen back and put some ink in it this time.

How do we do this?

Well, that's what the contents of this whole book are about. But here's where we have to start: we've got to come together. Yes, we've been a generation of anxiety, but what if we were a generation of community? What if we became IRL friends again? What if we were a generation willing to vulnerably connect? We may not necessarily have been taught how to do this (we've often been subversively taught to compete rather than unite) and the cards may be stacked against us, but I know it's possible.

I'm seeing it happen already. When I see people such as X González and David Hogg and their classmates, survivors of the Marjory Stoneman Douglas High School shooting, bring together over a million people in the March for Our Lives rally, I'm filled with hope. When I watch Greta Thunberg speaking up about climate change, I'm inspired. I'm even more inspired when she passes the mic to other activists and women of color, such as Disha Ravi from India, Vanessa Nakate from Uganda, and Mitzi Jonelle Tan from the Philippines, who have unfortunately, but not surprisingly, been robbed of airtime in the conversation.[25]

I'm equally heartened when I see my clients doing the work. Whether it's calling in a family member when they make a racist comment veiled as a "joke," wearing a bikini when you feel self-conscious that you don't have a "perfect" Instagram-filtered body, or going to the hospital because you don't feel like you can keep yourself safe—that all counts as doing the work.

I saw Nikita doing the work when she decided to accept herself fully. As we started to break the boundaries of what she saw as "okay" and "not okay," she realized that she could still identify as a Christian and expand her sexuality. For years, her faith had blocked her from accepting whom she felt genuinely attracted to, and, as a result, she would date man after man whom she felt no connection with. We started exploring different identities, and over time, she owned who she was as a queer woman. Stepping into herself fully, there was no shame or fear any longer. She was proud. The Nikita who hung her head low had been replaced by a woman who held her head high. She started dating people—people who were actually of interest to her and not just because she thought she "should" be seeing them. Before long, she was smoking, drinking, and spending less because she was too busy enjoying meeting new people. We both felt the power in the room when she told me one day, "Lauren . . . I'm actually really happy." It was undeniable—even to herself.

It takes bravery to make a different choice like Nikita did—to own your story. It's easier to stay home and tell ourselves it's too hard. We begin to think we don't deserve to hope for better. That's where Nikita was when I first saw her. But eventually, that place of desperation leads us to wonder whether there can be a way out. We start to consider that our pain may actually provide us with the path forward. Making a change in our lives can be so freaking uncomfortable and scary that sometimes our anxiety has to reach a fever pitch before we care enough to try something else.

So perhaps as you read this, you're at your breaking point. You're tired of the panic attacks that leave you shaking, sick, and exhausted. You're worn-out by the endless worrying about your future, your finances, your body, your dating life, your job, your grades—your whatever. You're fed up. I know it hurts. I've been there myself.

But here's the thing: you can be at your turning point. *Right now.*

I'm not promising that some of the stressors in your life will go away, but I can help you get your brain back. And it's all going to start with the choices you make. Staring at the news and lamenting at your screen isn't going to cut it. If we want things to be different, we have to start showing up differently. I'll say it again: **it's time to get our power back.** Whether it's starting to eat vegetarian to help protect our planet, intentionally spending time outside in greenery because of how it helps your mental health, or simply smiling at someone who is houseless rather than turning the other cheek, we've got to start reengaging.

And I have to tell you, it's not going to be comfortable or easy, but like many things in life, the good stuff rarely comes without some pain and sacrifice. We've gotten quite used to keeping ourselves in our enclosed spaces, making the world smaller for ourselves because we think it keeps us safe. Clearly, it doesn't.

We've got to start expanding ourselves again. We need to start asking questions about unconscious bias, even if that means we learn that we have our own and we feel ashamed (and, yep, we've all got biases whether or not we want to admit it). We need to start giving feedback to our managers and companies for how they can incorporate more mental health support, even if we fear they'll judge us for advocating for our well-being. We need to lean into conversations with people who are different from us, even if we or they say the wrong thing and we fumble our way through it. It's better to at least show up than to continue sitting out.

We've got to come back to each other. We've got to start caring about each other again.

Personal anxiety abates when we take ownership of our lives like Nikita did. It's when we accept what is—and we take a step forward anyway. This can happen on a singular level when we live a life aligned with our values (more on that in the next chapter). Whether it's going on a trip even though we have flight anxiety, or keeping up with our medical appointments even though we feel scared to go to the doctor, that's how we win the battle in our brains. Each of our struggles is unique but the strategy is the same: we face it.

But how to overcome the collective anxiety that has overtaken us on a societal level? It's accepting what is and coming together even more adamantly. It's the regathering in our roots and *knowing* one another again. We start to choose differently because we care. Because we see one another fully.

I call this *empowered acceptance*. It's a level of acceptance that is supercharged. It fuels the fight to make things better on a systemic level. It's a powerful holding of not just our own pain but the pain of our communities that allows us to sit with the discomfort in a new way. Empowered acceptance is empathy embodied and enacted.

And here's the thing—community does not have to mean commonality (something that I believe many of us can forget). We don't have to agree. In fact, the disparity in our opinions can make us further evaluate and achieve a more nuanced approach to these all-too-complex problems that can get oversimplified. I'm breaking this down in chapter 4.

I know this can all sound overwhelming. You may be thinking, "I can barely handle my own problems. How can I handle someone else's?" And that is what anxiety makes us think. It takes over all of our brain space.

And a warning: I'm now going to say something that you may not like.

Your anxiety is making you selfish. Your anxiety is making you obsess about what people thought of your outfit last night and whether the joke you told was funny. It stopped you from seeing that your friend was hinting that she's having a hard time at work or that she's struggling to conceive. You were too preoccupied to notice. You forgot to even ask how she's doing.

Your anxiety is telling you that people will judge you if you disagree with them, so you avoid talking about immigration policies or how to improve your work culture. You don't talk to your dad, even though you're losing sleep at night worrying about his drinking behavior. You don't want to make him mad. So instead, you talk about the weather and the latest trendy restaurant to try, all because you're not willing to be uncomfortable and risk anyone being upset with you.

Your anxiety is making you ruminate constantly about whether you're making the "right" choices. Whether this is the "best" job you could be at, whether now is the "perfect" time to have a baby, and whether you "should" have more friends. It's stopping you from seeing (and perhaps caring about) the pains of your colleagues, your friends, and the people you encounter on a daily basis.

It's not your fault. I'm not trying to shame you. That's just how powerful anxiety is. It pulls us down tight and makes us feel more and more alone in our heads. It tells us we're not strong enough, smart enough, funny enough, special enough, or brave enough so we need to keep things as safe and simple as possible. But this is all a lie.

The answer is coming out of the hole you've been in and reaching your hand out for help. And even though you may not feel like you have the strength, it's extending your hand to someone else to help them as well. When you can get beyond the haze of your own pain, you can see that there is healing in being a part of the solution for someone else.

These problems that we're all facing are so much bigger than ourselves and it's going to take all of us coming together to solve them. We're going to have to compromise and we may not always like the outcome. But where our healing truly lies is in our willingness to sit alongside one another again. We need to get out of our heads together and perhaps, like Forrest Gump, start eating a box of chocolates together on a park bench and telling each other our stories. Like Nikita told to me.

We don't have to do this alone, nor should we. Our healing comes from our collective caring that propels us forward. That's empowered acceptance. Give it a try.

CHAPTER THREE

WELCOME THE WAVES

LEARN HOW TO SURF RATHER THAN SINK IN YOUR TIDES

I'll be honest, some clients are a little harder to connect with. This can happen for a variety of reasons. Clients can have defenses that make them show up like porcupines with all their spikes up. Sometimes it's an assortment of jokes when things start to get serious, or it's a client's undeniable desire to *not* be in therapy, where they offer notable silences that even a therapist finds awkward. Other times it can happen when clients seem shut down to the process, appearing cut off from their emotions and offering stilted responses such as "I don't know" twenty times over. This is what Jacob was like at first.

Identifying as a cisgender, white, straight man, he was in his late twenties and had gone through two tours in Afghanistan before getting a corporate job. I could see how exhausted he looked. With bags under his eyes, he looked as if he could fall asleep in my office at any minute. His dazed silence gave everything away. He was past the point of emotionality. He had reached that stage of numbness where his eyes glazed over and his expression was blank. When I would ask what he was feeling, he'd often say, "Nothing," and the silence would sit between us.

As time went on, it became clear that Jacob had reached out to me because he was at a crossroads. He was mentally and emotionally drowning. He was consumed by guilt—he had proposed to his girlfriend and their wedding planning was in full swing. There was just one problem . . . he wasn't sure whether he actually wanted to marry her.

When I asked him how he ended up here, he told me, "I feel like I'm a parent in this relationship. I manage all of our finances. I clean up after her. I make all of our plans. She barely even says 'Thank you.'"

I then responded with the classic therapy question that is actually necessary in many cases: "And how does that make you feel, Jacob?"

"I feel like I'm never doing enough. I am finding myself resenting her. And yet . . . I'm stuck. It's too late to make a change."

I quietly answered, "Maybe it's never truly too late to get yourself out of a situation that isn't working."

And thus began our exploration of how Jacob found himself in the predicament he was in—and what he could do to find another path if he so desired. I make it clear in these cases that I have no judgment about what a client chooses to do ultimately—it is their decision and theirs alone.

What we learned is that with Jacob's anxious attachment style (where a person tends to be overly fearful of abandonment and being alone), he was afraid to let go of a relationship that had lasted for years after putting in so much time and work. He worried: what would it say about me if I were to walk away from this relationship? Jacob was a victim of the sunk cost fallacy—having already invested so much time, he wanted to believe that if he put in "just a little more," it might get better.[26]

I could see he was mentally treading. As he tried fervently to fight off his thoughts, images, and feelings that he didn't ultimately want this relationship, he was completely wearing himself out. He had learned how to ignore his body's and brain's cues that he was in distress. He would frequently stare off into space, sometimes for hours at a time. He would struggle to sleep, binge eat, and avoid having sex with his fiancée. As she kept pushing for their relationship to progress into marriage, he became more and more conflicted about what to do.

As this went on month after month, and eventually year after year, he succumbed to the belief that this was his "new normal." In fact, he had forgotten what it felt like to be happy. When I asked him what brought him joy, he responded with "I don't even know anymore."

His brain fed him a constant dose of myths, including that he was a failure, that his relationship struggling was entirely his fault, and that if he were a better partner and worked harder, his relationship would improve. At his core, he believed he was unlovable. He was approaching his partnership from the mindset that he'd never find someone whom he felt he actually had a connection with.

Does this sound familiar to you? As is often the case with anxiety, we settle for mediocrity because we think we're lucky to get anything at all. So many of us, like Jacob, exhaust ourselves with an endless stream of negative thoughts like this. Perhaps you resonated with the examples just shared from Jacob's mindset, but in case you need some others, here are just a few more things you may be mentally treading against:

- Thoughts that you are a failure or that you're terrible at your job
- Images of you embarrassing yourself or losing control somehow (e.g., getting sick in public, breaking or spilling something and people looking at you, or letting one rip accidentally)
- Feelings of inadequacy in your relationships and believing it's only a matter of time until everyone leaves you
- Believing that you are "broken" because you feel anxious or depressed
- Ruminating over the future and your perceived inability to cope

Do any of these land for you? We start spiraling based on the messages our brains send us. And yes, I said *send*. Whether you like it or not, your brain has an automatic mail delivery system where it sometimes delivers helpful information, and other times it gives you nothing but spam. Where it gets confusing is in trying to filter out the helpful data from the junk pile, as the brain's mail person delivers them simultaneously. Our anxious brains can get overwhelmed by this, and we may try to block the process entirely.

The fancy term for this: "disassociation." Dissociation is when we can feel disconnected from our minds, bodies, feelings, memories, and identity.[27] You may have experienced this momentarily when your eyes have trouble focusing or you feel like you're out of your body for a few moments. For some, it can last for a much more extended period of time, developing into depersonalization/derealization disorder, where people feel disconnected from their physicality or their surroundings for hours, days, months, or more.

Here's the thing, though. Just as you can't control your spam folder filling up, you are not responsible for the thoughts or images that pop up in your brain. Sometimes, the mind gives us ideas or pictures that we'd really rather not have. Some are rooted in reality, like the possibility for Jacob that his relationship would end, and some are far-fetched and highly unlikely. For example—and get ready for this—I'm guessing you don't want to imagine peeing your pants in public. Or your pet getting hit by a car. Or getting fired from your job this week.

Okay, I'll stop before you really start hating me. But truthfully, that was the PG version. I bet your mind has come up with a lot worse than that.

I say these things because chances are that your brain has already been giving you these thoughts and images anyway. It looks different for each person, but ultimately, our brains love to introduce all kinds of wacky, unpleasant, and worst-case-scenario thoughts and images that make us do a double take on ourselves. That is simply what the brain does. While there are findings indicating a wide range in the number of thoughts we have in a given day, at a minimum, the brain churns out about six thousand thoughts a day.[28] Better yet: most of those thoughts are considered to be negative in nature and repetitive in context.

This is how the brain has held power over you. Each time an upsetting idea or image pops up, you may have said to yourself, "What's wrong with you?! You're so [disgusting, weird, stupid, messed-up]—how could you have had that thought?" You start worrying that it's *just* you who's had these thoughts, and before you know it, you've got a classic case of what we call meta-worrying.

What's meta-worrying? It's when you start worrying about how much you're worrying. Sound familiar? You notice yourself obsessing about that interview, that date, or that conversation (from seven years ago), and before you know it, you're freaked out because, really—you shouldn't be this freaked out . . . right?

Then start the mental cues: "But why am I so worried?" "What does this mean that I am so worried?" "Is this a sign because I am so worried?" Or the best: "I'm noticing that I haven't been as worried lately. Perhaps I should be worrying about that . . ."

Notice a key word there: "should."

As the saying goes, when it comes to anxiety, so many of us are should-ing on ourselves. We internally scold ourselves for something we have literally no control over—our minds.

I don't mean for that to unnerve you. I say it to help ground you. Because once you know that it's not your fault that you feel anxious or that you have uncomfortable, scary, or gross thoughts sometimes, that's when you take the wheel again. That's when you start to actually feel like you have some control in your life again.

The brain is a wild and free agent. It comes up with all kinds of odd, quirky, frustrating thoughts. But that's just the brain being its true self. In fact, the brain loves to come up with the worst-case scenario, where we lose our job, we find out our partner is cheating on us, and we all die from a huge meteor hitting the earth. Okay, I'll stop with the examples.

The great news is that we are not the sum of our thoughts. If we were, we honestly wouldn't make much sense. A thought is simply a thought—it doesn't mean it has actual truth.

Let me say that again in case you missed it: *a thought is just a thought.*

It doesn't mean it's valid, real, or accurate. It could be—but it might not be, either. Starting to get curious (and even a little cautious) about the data your brain is trying to give you is going to help you stay afloat in your water that much longer. The sooner we can realize this, the more liberated we are to engage with our experiences and relationships. We are no longer a victim to the mind and what it's trying to tell us. In other words, the jig is up, and the brain can get in line because you're no longer buying the BS.

WHY POSITIVE THINKING CAN TAKE A WALK

Speaking of BS, I'm calling out positive thinking, changing your thoughts, or "training" your brain. Because as much as we may want to control our minds, our brains can be unruly. That's why, for example, mindfulness is a *practice* that's about building awareness of our thoughts—it's never an act of mastery.

You may have found yourself especially frustrated because you've tried all the "brain hacks" to change your thinking and it's just not cutting it. People can get into some really dangerous territory because they have been told that if only they could "think positively," they would feel better. Or they have been told that they can pray it away, ignore it, or change it (and you know how this goes thanks to meta-worrying); that tends to only amplify the thoughts and corresponding distress when we can't in fact change our thoughts.

So, let me say this loud and clear: there's nothing wrong with you if you have anxious or obsessive thoughts. We all have them from time to time. For some, it just happens to be a little (or a lot) more frequent. This isn't by happenstance, either. There are literally mechanisms in the brain that contribute to people experiencing ruminating thoughts. Specifically, with obsessive-compulsive disorder (OCD), we see overactivity in the orbitofrontal cortex (OFC), anterior cingulate cortex (ACC),

and caudate nucleus.[29] So, while you may be feeling like you're responsible for giving yourself these upsetting thoughts that just won't seem
to go away, it's actually your brain doing the work for you. How kind.

Now, I know. I'm going to put it simply: this plain *sucks*. This is the
part of the acceptance work that's the struggle. Many of us go through
a period where we resent our minds, compare ourselves to others, and
say, "Why me? Why do others seem so unbothered by their minds and
I'm over here losing sleep, second-guessing everything, and feeling miserable?" If you feel like it's unfair, it is. Just as some people are not able
to use their legs to run or their eyes to see, some people have minds that
auto-populate with indecision, morbidity, and catastrophe. But just as
a person does not have a choice in the matter of their legs or eyes, the
same goes for how the brain functions as well. Thankfully there are
approaches we can take regarding how we respond to these thoughts,
but at an entry point, we have to acknowledge and accept when the
brain feels like a relentless tyrant inside ourselves.

When we come to terms with this reality, it's common to go through
a grieving process. I've seen it with many clients, especially those who
have had decades-long battles with anxiety and/or depression. It makes
sense that we feel this sadness. If we could make the anxiety go away,
we would, wouldn't we? And we've tried valiantly, too. Just in 2019
alone, we spent $225 billion on mental health services, an increase of
52 percent since 2009.[30] Many of us cycle through therapists, medica-
tions, and the latest treatment fad, hoping that it will "cure" us finally.

But struggling sometimes is what it means to be human—what it
means to have a brain. When we can allow ourselves to feel the sadness
that the brain hands us, we can learn how to cope with it. We're no longer living in a space of denial where we doubt ourselves. Instead, we're
acknowledging it for what it is.

Now, at first this may feel like defeat. That by accepting your anxiety,
you're losing the battle in your brain. But it's actually winning the war.

I get what it's like all too well. Anxiety has tried to rule my life in
so many ways, but I would say none more so than with respect to my

decision about whether to start a family. Anxiety has told me, "You wouldn't be a good mother—you have no experience." It's also tried to tell me, "You like control too much. Babies are the definition of a lack of control." And my favorite, "A baby would change everything. Why would you want to mess everything up?" Really fun being inside my head, right?

It doesn't help that my experience with emetophobia has added on some nice excuses for why I could never become a parent. After all, when you're basically deathly afraid of vomit, who would willingly enter into potentially nine months of morning sickness (yep, you know I've researched hyperemesis gravidarum, which is when you basically throw up every day of your pregnancy and sometimes get hospitalized because it's so bad) to then have a child who could projectile-vomit on you (and at you) at any given moment? So you can see that as I'm now in my thirties, this tape has played for a while.

With these thoughts floating in my head and churning in my stomach, it all becomes so confusing.

Even more confusing is that anxiety often makes us want to be everything to everyone. It tells us to conform—to wash ourselves away entirely. It tells us to not stand out, speak up, or share our true identities. It tells us that we are only loved and accepted when we agree and go with the crowd. As someone who has straddled that line, I can tell you it's much better to be on the side where you embrace yourself fully. And counterintuitively, people tend to connect with you even more when they see you allowing yourself to be true to you.

It's okay to own and accept who you are. I know your anxiety (and especially your perfectionism) may have told you for years that no one loves you, that you're ugly, or that you're an idiot. It doesn't mean there is actual validity to these thoughts. Once we break this association, the guilt and shame can start to go away. We begin to learn that you may have the thought that you are stupid, but it does not mean you are actually stupid. You may have the thought that you're not creative, but that doesn't mean you're not actually creative.

Now you may be asking, "But Lauren ... what if my thought is actually true?" And sure, I'm not telling you to invalidate yourself completely. But could it be that you're being way harder on yourself than you would with anyone else? Could there be evidence that you may in fact not be the ultimate failure or loser you've told yourself that you are? You get to decide what you believe, who you want to be, and how you want to live your life. There is no number of anxious thoughts in your brain that can ever stop you from being the person you want to become. So, while you can't control the thoughts, you can control what you do with them. How you respond to your thoughts is where you get your power back.

This concept was a game changer for Jacob. Once he began to learn that his thoughts about being unlovable and incapable of making change were not absolute truths, he was able to regain control in his waters again. He was no longer a victim of the tides of his mind. He could start responding in all-new ways that grounded him after years of feeling lost at sea. Some pretty powerful things were about to happen.

A NEW WAVE TO RIDE:
Who is that person you want to be? What would you wear, say, listen to, and do if anxiety weren't stopping you?

YOU DON'T HAVE TO FIGHT SO HARD
I'm guessing that this book has brought up a lot for you already, and just reading this far may have been exhausting. You may have already felt mentally drained before you picked up this book. You may have tried just about everything—therapy, medication, retreats, doctors' visits—and the anxiety is still there. Many of us put our lives on pause, hoping the anxiety will magically go away. That's what Jacob did, keeping himself in a stagnant relationship for nearly a decade. We can waste years, losing opportunities with our careers, our dating lives, and our friendships, because we hope that we'll *eventually* feel better.

Here's where I'm sorry to tell you—staying at home and waiting is not going to solve the problem. In fact, it's only going to make it worse. Every time we pull back, we give our anxiety a penny. Those pennies add up. Before we know it, our anxiety is rich in the bank and we're broke in spirit (and maybe actual cash from trying to throw money at our problems). We feel weaker and weaker each time anxiety wins. Before long, anxiety has convinced us that we're *just not ready* to get out there.

So, let me say it to you straight: **you're never going to be ready**.

You're never going to feel prepared enough to go out on that date. You're never going to feel qualified enough to apply for that job. You're never going to feel like you have enough money before you have a baby. You're never going to believe that you have enough followers to feel like people care about what you have to say.

The truth is, no one is ever fully ready, but I can guarantee that you are more ready than you realize. I'm not saying to fully fake it until you make it, but I am saying that maybe it's time to start putting yourself out there before you're 100 percent prepared.

One of the biggest ways to break through the weight of anxiety is to be brave enough to ask for what you want. This is when we're willing to ask for a raise, invite someone on a date, and apply for that position that feels like a long shot.

I've seen this happen in my own life. You see, if there's one thing I try to cling to, even with anxiety, it's a sense of fearlessness—especially when it comes to people. That doesn't mean I don't hold fear; it just means that I try to care less about the fear than I do my future. Case in point: Who do you think asked her now-husband out on the first date? Yours truly. Thirteen years later, I'm glad I did.

There's so much that can happen in your life when you're willing to be uncomfortable. Anxiety is going to tell you at every juncture that you can't do it—that you should just play it safe. But safety rarely secures the life you're looking to live.

I hope reading this will get you excited to put yourself out there. Screw being fully prepared. No one ever is. What matters is that you give it a go. Trust that you will figure it out along the way. I'm not asking you to go to the finish line, I'm just asking you to start. The finish line will come in good time, but you won't get there if you're not willing to take that first step.

For Jacob, his first step moved him in a different direction. His bravery looked like saying aloud for the first time (though he had been thinking it for so long): "I don't think I want to be in this relationship anymore." Within seconds, that courage became transformative, and he saw his anxiety abate for the first time in years. That's how powerful facing our fear head-on can be. Life-changing, in fact.

A NEW WAVE TO RIDE:

What first step can you take? What have you been saying that you're not ready for that you actually might be?

THE DREADED DIVING BOARD

I know this is all so scary. The idea of this kind of vulnerability may leave you sweating straight through your shirt right now. You may be saying, "That sounds nice, but you don't understand. I'm just not ready." And that may be the case. We have to respect where we sit. But can we gently nudge ourselves to take a step? Or a jump? Here's one of my favorite metaphors that I like to use in session with my clients. As you read it, think about where you stand in the context of this example.

I want you to imagine yourself staring up at a thirty-three-foot diving board. You can feel your stomach dropping already, but you start to climb the ladder. You may notice that your knees are buckling, your hands are clammy, and it's starting to feel hard to breathe. As you get to the top of the diving board, you look down and start to feel a little wobbly. You may mutter an expletive or two under your breath because, dang—this is higher up than you realized. As you stand on the edge, you look down at the water below.

This is the moment.

Do you jump in? Do you take that leap of faith? Or do you step back and feel the board tremble?

Whether or not you've stood on a high dive before, we've all been there before, figuratively speaking. It's that feeling right before we get onstage to give a speech, before we tell someone we like them, or before we tell someone they've hurt us. It was that moment for Jacob when he said aloud that he wanted to break up with his fiancé.

With each jump, we realize something profound. We learn that we can swim. We learn once we hit the water that we're capable. We see that we are no longer a victim of our fear. We also start to see that the feeling of vulnerability doesn't last forever. When we go for it, there's a sense of bravery that no one can ever take away from us. We see in that moment that we are more powerful than our anxiety.

So where are you in this narrative? Are you jumping in or are you slowly stepping away from the edge of the board?

The problem is, when it comes to anxiety, many of us sit on the ledge and just look down. We wonder, "What if I can't swim?" "What if I hit my head?" "What if it's scary?" "What if the water's cold?"

Here's the translation: What if they reject me? What if I fail? What if I look like an idiot?

What if? What if? What if? Let's break these "what-ifs" down and reframe them as what they may actually represent:

- **"What if they reject me?"**
  - **The reframe:** Rejection is actually a great gift and a time-saver. Rejection helps us identify the people and experiences that may not be for us so that we can get on to finding the right opportunities and connections instead.
- **"What if I fail?"**
  - **The reframe:** You'll learn invaluable information each time you fail. It will sharpen your skills for next time around. "Failure" is a sign that you are showing up for

your life and putting yourself out there so that you can learn.

- **"What if I look like an idiot?"**
  - ○ **The reframe:** If someone judges you for putting yourself out there, that says more about their own insecurities. Yes, being a beginner may mean you look silly or even ignorant. Trust that others will have compassion for your learning process and give yourself major credit for leaning into the growth process.

If you're feeling stuck, you need to ask yourself this question: "When I look back on my life, do I want to have lived bravely, jumping off my diving board, or do I want to have stayed where I was?"

When we think about where we stand, this is ultimately highlighting the difference between five seconds of courage and five minutes or five years of regret.

We've all been there before. Whether you literally got on a diving board and then turned around or you passed on a potentially great opportunity, you may find yourself wondering, *"What if I had been brave?"* Ironic, isn't it, that the "what-if" question is coming back around.

So . . . what if? What if you were bold enough to believe you had a chance? What if you just went for it? What if you saw what was on the other side?

I watched Jacob climb up his metaphorical diving board in our work together. He started out trembling, afraid of what he would find. But it was when he took that leap of faith, when he told his fiancée that he was going to move out of their apartment, that he reported a wave of immense relief wash over him. Yes, he felt sad that his relationship hadn't worked. But more than anything, he felt a profound sense of peace as he was able to finally take action. Something amazing happened after that, too: Jacob started to feel a new jolt of confidence that he hadn't felt since college. There was about to be a whole new Jacob, both in session and out.

THE SPRINGS THAT HELP YOU TAKE THE JUMP FORWARD

Personally, I never want the "what-ifs" to rule me. That is why I am so committed to not letting my anxiety run my life—or yours, for that matter.

One of the best ways we can sit with our anxiety is knowing what we value. Knowing what matters to you is the grounding you need when your legs are jelly and everything in your mind is saying, "Turn back now."

We need our values not only to guide us, but to help us sit through the pain of life. It's a lot easier to stay at home, continue in our ho-hum relationship, and keep up with the monotony, even if it's not working for us. When we're lacking a clear definition of what our values are, we can find ourselves making all kinds of excuses for why "now just isn't a good time." Life keeps handing you opportunities and instead of listening to the offer, your anxiety tells you no every time.

But here's the thing: pain often holds tremendous worth. The pain, though uncomfortable, is not something that we need to be afraid of and run from forever. Is it painful to break up with your partner of ten years? Heck yes. Is it hard to quit your job and pursue a new career path instead? Certainly. Does it suck to admit that your friendship is no longer working and it's time to end it? Of course. But are making those changes worth it? Straight from the mouth of a therapist who has heard it from hundreds of clients: YES. Let me say this loud and clear: **we need to choose values induction over pain reduction**.

You *can* sit with the pain. Trust me. I know you don't believe it— but most of the time, you can. And that's why knowing what your values are is everything. If you are clear on what you care about, you're going to be able to endure the pain of change because you know it is moving you toward the life that you aspire to have. When you're clear on what's core for you, the pain isn't just bearable; it may even be worth it.

Let's put this into context. Let's say you value intimacy, connection, and passion and you're in a relationship that looks great on paper but is missing all three of those core values. Though it's going to hurt like heck when you end that relationship because your values aren't being met, those same values will ground you when you're crying in your car, wondering how you'll ever get over the heartbreak. Though it will still suck, you'll feel proud of yourself for choosing your values over convenience or reputation. If you value creativity, independence, and leadership, you're going to be able to endure that tough conversation with your boss to tell them that this job isn't working for you anymore. If you value humor, risk-taking, and fun but you have a strong case of social anxiety, you'll be that much more inclined to get on the stage for your stand-up routine because you know what matters the most to you.

Values can be our compass that helps us know what to do when we've got a tough decision to make. Whether you are indecisive (which is one of the hallmarks of anxiety), tend to make decisions to appease others (hello, people pleasers!), or make decisions out of haste because the anticipation is too much for you, your values can recenter you. When you've got a choice to make about starting a new job, moving to a different city, or, yes, even getting a pet, ask yourself honestly, "How do my values align or not align with this decision that I'm considering?" If your values are absent from the option you're planning to choose, that gives you some helpful data that anxiety may be inserting itself in the narrative as a "value."

Now, some of you may be thinking, "But what about when my values conflict?! What about when I value challenge but I also value safety and comfort? What if I value dependability but I also seek spontaneity? What if I'm considering taking on a new promotion but I also want to protect my mental health and self-care? What if I want to start a family but I'm just getting started with this next step in my career?"

I've got two things for you here.

One, implement the 10/10/10 rule. Ask yourself: "If I were to make my decision in this way, how would I feel about it ten minutes from now? How about ten months from now? What about ten years from now?" Notice if any feelings of regret, curiosity, anticipation, or anything else bubbles up for you. This can help you see the bigger picture to evaluate whether your values are integrated or anxiety is trying to steal the show.

The other point I want to stress that may surprise you: **life can be long**.

I know—you probably weren't expecting that. We're always told that life is short and that we need to make the most of it. Unfortunately, for us anxious folks, we have taken that message reallyyyyy close to heart (and to the head). We feel like we need to do everything NOW and we need to do it at our absolute best. We'll forgo sleep, meals, and relationships just to get to the bottom line of our next goal.

If we're lucky, though, we've got a lot of life to live. You don't have to do everything in your twenties, thirties, or forties. You don't have to be a smashing success before you finish college. Shocker: you don't have to be a smashing success ever because maybe, just maybe, your worth isn't defined by your accomplishments. Life is more than checked boxes. The people who matter most to you are not bullet points that can be added to your résumé.

So, given that, ask yourself what matters the most to you long term, especially when you're conflicted. When you look back on your life, how do you hope you will have spent your time? Yes, you may be torn about whether you should advance in your career or focus on becoming a parent. But perhaps there can be both. Perhaps there is a time and a season for each. Perhaps they can coexist—even though it won't be perfect (and that's okay!).

If there can't be room for each, can we integrate some acceptance into our choice as we know that our decision, though imperfect and painful, is rooted deeply in what we care about the most—our values?

Life can get so confusing and when we're bombarded with choices, we can feel paralyzed. Our values can be so powerful that they may be enough to see us through our anxiety that muddles our waters. They're the impetus that drives us through all the worry and doubt.

There aren't many rules when it comes to values. In fact, I always say that there are no such things as "bad values," so long as they do not physically harm you or someone else. That may mean your values may emotionally hurt someone (case in point: ending a relationship that isn't aligning with your values, even though it will upset the other person). So as we go through Jacob's story, I invite you to notice any biases or judgments that may come up for you and hold them with a gentle curiosity as you try to empathize with Jacob's perspective.

When someone is struggling to identify their values, it can be helpful to start with a person's history and how they identify intersectionally. For Jacob, we looked at how his life as a straight, cisgender man, raised in Louisiana in a religious and conservative family, was informing his perspective. We explored how he held some traditionalist ideas of masculinity and religiosity that were making him feel guilty for not being "even more committed" to the relationship than he already had been. While he had given it his all and was miserable in the process, he felt that as an adult man, he "should" continue in his unhappy relationship from a place of honor and respect for his partner—even if the love was absent. We were also able to note how his history in the marines played into his values of loyalty and dedication, no matter what. As we explored this, we were able to identify what Jacob's "should" values were versus his actual values.

Our "should" values are often societal in nature. We hold our parents', our teachers', and even strangers' opinions on what we're "supposed" to value as the standard to strive for in life. Jacob felt like he "should" value commitment, honor, and dedication—particularly in his relationship—and that is why he trudged along for years in a lifeless partnership for the facade of public and familial approval.

But eventually we were able to sit with what Jacob actually valued. He noted that vulnerability, reciprocity, and respect in a relationship were crucial for him—and they were missing at present. It was upon this realization that many of his true values were absent, including that of personal happiness, that he found the courage to ask his fiancée to call off the wedding with him. The relief he felt in taking this step was tremendous; at the same time, he acknowledged that he felt awful that his ex-fiancée was, understandably, upset. Even though it was a major shift in his life, he felt a sense of alignment—which had been absent for years—because he clarified his values for the first time.

Now, you may have noticed your own feelings come up as you read what happened for Jacob. You may have felt like Jacob "gave up" on his relationship or that he's a selfish asshole, as he put his happiness before his commitment to her. This may be an indication that commitment is a top value for you. We all have different values that matter more to us, and that's okay. The important thing is that we are honest with one another about where we stand while still being respectful of the values that others hold.

When we're dishonest (or lying to ourselves) about what we value, this is when we can get into some dark territory. It's also when we can hurt others the most. In fact, Jacob recognized that by minimizing his values and trying to stay in the relationship, he was actually disrespecting and dishonoring his fiancée even more. What he realized, though, was that it was better to be true to both of them *now* than wait for years, coexisting in an unhappy relationship just to keep the peace.

Part of why we end up hurting ourselves and others is because many of us simply don't know what our values are. We may hear the term "values" come up in conversation frequently, but it's rare that we've ever been guided through a process to define what our personal values actually are. This is how we can feel like we're getting caught up in a rip current in our lives, because we don't have our values to serve as our lighthouse.

One of my favorite things to do with clients is to go through a values card sorting exercise to help them get clear on what their top ten values are. We're about to do something similar. When you look at the following list of words, you're likely going to say that you like most of these words. After all, most values have some kind of positive connotation attached. But as you go through this list, ask yourself: "What values can I not live without? What values give my life a sense of meaning? What values do I want to align with, so much so that even others would be able to recognize them in me?"

WELCOME THE WAVES

START BY CIRCLING THE TOP TWENTY VALUES YOU IDENTIFY WITH:

Acceptance	Fitness	Originality
Achievement	Flexibility	Passion
Adventure	Forgiveness	Patience
Aesthetics	Freedom	Patriotism
Affection	Generosity	Peace
Ambition	Genuineness	Physical health
Authenticity	Gratitude	Play
Belonging	Growth	Pleasure
Challenge	Honesty	Popularity
Comfort	Hope	Power
Commitment	Humility	Practicality
Community	Humor	Protection
Cooperation	Imagination	Providing
Courage	Independence	Rationality
Courtesy	Integrity	Responsibility
Creativity	Intimacy	Risk-taking
Credibility	Justice	Resilience
Curiosity	Knowledge	Romance
Dedication	Leadership	Security
Dependability	Learning	Self-control
Duty	Legacy	Self-improvement
Efficiency	Leisure	Service
Empathy	Love	Social justice
Excitement	Mastery	Spirituality
Expertise	Mentorship	Spontaneity
Exploration	Moderation	Stability
Faithfulness	Novelty	Success
Fame	Nurturing	Tradition
Family	Openness	Tolerance
Financial success	Order	Wisdom

ADD ANY ADDITIONAL VALUES NOT LISTED ABOVE THAT RESONATE
FOR YOU:

_____

_____

_____

_____

_____

LIST ANY VALUES THAT BRING UP A NEGATIVE CONNOTATION FOR
YOU AND WRITE OUT WHY:

_____

_____

_____

_____

_____

_____

ARE THERE ANY VALUES THAT YOU FEEL SOCIETY OR OTHERS ARE
TELLING YOU THAT YOU "SHOULD" VALUE, EVEN THOUGH YOU
DON'T IDENTIFY WITH THEM? IF SO, LIST HERE AND EXPLAIN:

_____

_____

_____

_____

_____

_____

BASED ON THE TOP TWENTY WORDS YOU CIRCLED, RANK YOUR TOP TEN VALUES, ALONG WITH WHY EACH VALUE MATTERS TO YOU:

1. _____

2. _____

3. _____

4. _____

5. _____

6. _____

7. _____

8. _____

9. _____

10. _____

Now here's the thing: I see so many situations where people have let their anxiety win and their values lose. Where they have said to themselves that it's just *not worth it* to go on a blind date, to confront a racist family member, or to go out to a great new restaurant by themselves because they don't want to be uncomfortable. These examples widely vary but there's a common theme.

Those are days when team anxiety takes a *W* and our values take an *L*. I'm not here for it.

When I think of this in the context of becoming a parent myself, I think about how anxiety could easily win this battle in my life. The fear of my child throwing up in my hair while I'm driving or the idea that I'll take up permanent residence at château porcelain for nine—but really ten—months could easily be enough for me to walk away.

But I'll be damned if my anxiety makes that decision for me. I may not become a mother because I decide that I want to dedicate more time to my career, or that I want to travel more, or that I just plain don't want to—but I will not let my anxiety make that choice for me. Letting my fear, especially my irrational fear with my phobia, determine the outcome of something as monumental as having children in my life is just not something I'm willing to agree to. To me, a brave life that is aligned with my values is the one I want to always choose instead of the life that is indebted to an avoidance of anxiety.

Powerful things happened for Jacob when he reassessed his true values. Simply put: I started to see Jacob become fully alive. More than anything, I saw his eyes brighten for the first time. That glazed look that he had in the beginning had transformed into an animated face that was seeing the world clearly for the first time in a long while. Jacob was starting to see in color.

WHAT HAPPENS WHEN YOU JUMP IN . . . OR DON'T

Think of all the times you have been brave enough to dive in. I guarantee, every time you've made a choice in your life out of courage, rather than fear, something transformative has happened. An incredible person may have come into your life. You may have created something magnificent for others to enjoy. You may have learned something invaluable that no one can ever take away. Major bonus: that anxiety that was trying to stop you also probably got a lot smaller. Every time we face a fear, anxiety loses its power, brick by brick.

We all know the opposite feeling, though. It's that feeling when we don't jump off the board and we turn around to climb back down the ladder. But let's be honest, when we crawl back down, internally, it feels so good for a split second, doesn't it? That relief of avoidance is tremendous. It's that text where we cancel our plans for the night, the day we call in sick when we're totally fine, and that moment when we say, "Count me out." It can feel glorious.

But what about after that initial moment of relief? We start to hear that little voice in our head say, "But what if you did it? *What if* you jumped in the pool?" There's that darn "what-if" again.

But sometimes, we'll never know. Some of us try to go through life never getting in the pool. We've convinced ourselves that we can't swim.

Now, I'm not trying to guilt or shame you. Sometimes we do have to pull back. Sometimes the board is too high and if we took that leap, we'd end up with a broken leg. This is where you need to have some self-compassion. Sometimes you do need to say no and walk off the diving board. That is totally okay. We've got to take a break sometimes, and when you do pull back, be kind to yourself in that process. Being brave and vulnerable takes a lot of mental (and physical) energy, and sometimes we simply don't have it. Shaming ourselves isn't going to make it any easier to jump into the pool next time.

However, we need to get back on the board when we can (and likely before we're fully ready). It's not meant to be easy. We've got to be intentional about giving ourselves that little nudge to climb up because every time we pull back, it gets harder and harder to jump off.

Take the example of someone who wants to find a partner and is actively dating. At first, it feels scary to ask someone whether you can kiss them, right? They may reject you and it could be cringey if they're not vibing with you. But if you let this fear hold you back, the bar lowers each time. Before you know it, it feels too scary to even go on a dating app and simply text someone. We start to doubt our abilities and sooner or later, we're in a long-term relationship with Netflix, Door-Dash, and online shopping.

You can see how it cascades quickly because fear can have that kind of power over our lives. Fear can be contagious, and it can make us feel weak. When we walk away from ourselves, we have chosen the comfort of familiarity instead of the growth that comes with the unknown. This is what happened for Jacob as he let years go by in a miserable relationship because he didn't want to endure the potential discomfort of making a change.

And our brains can be so good at coming up with excuses. Avoidance is sneaky in that way, but I assure you with baby steps, you will see yourself becoming braver and braver. You can handle a higher and higher diving board. This is because you begin to learn that each time you jump, you can swim and navigate the waters you're in. You can handle the vulnerability in the free fall because you know it will get you to the destination that matters to you. It will bring you back to your values and connect you to the life that you want to be living. That's worth the jump every time. And before you know it, you'll be that kid who can't stop climbing up and jumping off the board because you're having so much fun that you practically forget that you were afraid to begin with.

That's not to say it will always be easy. For Jacob, he still worried that his old patterns would spring back up in the new relationship he was in. He felt a crushing amount of guilt for leaving the old relationship, and we had to continue to process it for months after. After all, with values induction often comes pain. I would be lying if I said that the progress for Jacob was linear—it never is for any of us. But the important thing is that he realized what mattered to him. He began living his life in a way that felt true to him. He finally jumped in the pool—and was seeing that he could swim after all. I want you to know that you can, too.

CHAPTER FOUR

EMBRACING THE RIDE EVEN WHEN YOUR OCEAN IS COLD AND SCARY

~~~~~~

It's not uncommon for first-time clients to bring a family member or friend to their first session of therapy (I invite you to do the same if you're hesitant). Luís brought his sister with him, and it was hard to tell who was more nervous. With drops of sweat building on his brow, he glanced up when I called his name in the waiting room. Identifying as a gay, Catholic, Mexican cisgender male, he told me that he wasn't sure about this whole therapy thing. I tried my best to alleviate his worries, but I could tell the shame cycle had been spinning for a long time with Luís. He seemed embarrassed to be there—like he had failed because he made this appointment. I happened to see it as the opposite. I'm always inspired when clients have the strength to reach out. I hoped that I'd get a chance to help him see that.

As we went through the intake process, it became clear that Luís had been struggling with OCD for quite some time. While you can have just obsessions or compulsions to meet diagnostic criteria, Luís was experiencing both. And while some clients have a specific set of triggers, Luís's symptoms ran the gamut from circling the block out of fear that he hit someone with his car to a fear of germs on the toilet seat and the obsessive thought (content warning) of stabbing his father.

If you're having a strong reaction to reading that, it's understandable. But just imagine your brain being pelted by these unwanted thoughts and images on a daily basis all the time—that is OCD in a nutshell. I know that for many of you reading this book, you don't have to imagine this. What I just described is all too real for you. I've had many clients say it feels like their brain is "on fire." Perhaps yours has been too and you're looking for the fire extinguisher.

OCD always pulls on my heartstrings. It can be incredibly painful, and I could tell that Luís was worn-out by his battle. Among the fears previously listed, he was also petrified of saying the "wrong" thing. He would scroll through his phone meticulously, worrying that he said or did something that would incriminate him, make him lose his job, or ostracize him from society. He would analyze conversations with friends and avoided ever sharing his opinion for fear that someone would disagree with him and rage against him. Even though he couldn't think of anything that would be damaging to his reputation (and was truly one of the kindest and softest-spoken souls you could ever meet), he fretted over the possibility that he could have done something that would derail his life.

Now, whether or not you're relating to Luís's experience, I believe this content is likely still of value—OCD diagnosis or not. While OCD is in a section of the *DSM-5* that's separate from other anxiety disorders, most of us can relate to experiencing obsessive thoughts to some degree, and wanting to engage in some compulsive behaviors to make ourselves feel better. To meet full criteria for diagnosis, a person needs to engage in obsessions or compulsions for at least an hour each day and/or experience significant distress socially, occupationally, or in other areas of functioning.[31] While only about 1 percent of the US population meets the full diagnostic criteria for OCD (equating to about 2 to 3 million adults at any given time), we can each identify, if not empathize, with the framework of how obsessions and compulsions work.[32]

OCD can look and feel many different ways. It's not just the typical "germophobia" that people reference. It's different from obsessive-compulsive personality disorder, where we see folks fixate on organization, orderliness, and perfectionism in a way that feels necessary for them. OCD is what we call ego-dystonic, meaning that the person typically *does not* like having the symptoms and desperately wants them to go away. Even though people may say "I'm so OCD" when they're expressing their desire to have a well-organized space or schedule, those with true OCD usually find their symptoms incredibly distressing and even debilitating. In fact, those with OCD often feel either tremendous shame in disclosing their thoughts, or the need to repeatedly check in with others for validation that they're "okay."

OCD can manifest in many ways as well. It can include a particular theme that a person will fixate on, though it's not uncommon that folks will have various triggers that can change over time as life stressors and situations evolve.

Let's cover some of these. None of this is meant to be diagnostic, nor are these subsets noted in the *DSM-5*. This is a tool to provide further clarity and to help you know that you're not alone if you experience any of these thoughts and/or compulsions.

COMMON FEARS OF OCD:

- **Harm-based:** This includes violent thoughts and a fear of carrying out violent actions. While we all experience disturbing thoughts and images from time to time, we can usually shrug them off, saying to ourselves, "Well, that was odd . . ." And then we move on. With this form of OCD, though, you may fixate on these harm-based obsessions and ruminate about "what it means" that you had these thoughts or images in the first place. You might wonder, "What if I really did kill that person and just don't know it?" It's not uncommon that you ask family or friends about your behavior (e.g., "Are you sure I didn't do anything wrong?"), and you might avoid people whom you fear you could harm.

- **Sexual orientation/gender identification:** With this subset of OCD, you might wonder whether you are "actually" gay or straight or trans or cisgender, among other identities. It's not always the different sexual orientation or gender identification that is distressing (although it could be for that particular person); it's more so the inability to put oneself in a box. This lack of 100 percent certainty is what usually causes the distress. As a result, you may avoid looking at or engaging with others who may activate the obsessive thought. Alternatively, you may "test it out" by looking at people who are triggering to see whether you notice yourself having a physical response. A big part of the treatment is working to destigmatize identity (if this is part of the distress) while also building tolerance for uncertainty.

- **Pedophilia:** Highly stigmatized, this can be one of the most painful forms of OCD. This is when the person worries that they *could* be a pedophile, though they have never engaged in any of these behaviors. Because pedophilia is a serious crime, those with this form of OCD can experience a great deal of distress and may struggle to seek support because of the high level of shame associated with it.

- **Relationship-based:** This can include everything from wondering whether your partner is the "right" person for you, worrying they may leave you, or doubting whether your partner actually loves you. This form of OCD can feel like being at the Cheesecake Factory: it's hard to decide what to pick on the menu and then once you do, even if you like your meal, you wonder whether you should have ordered something that could have tasted just a *little* better.

- **"Just right":** This can manifest in several different ways, but it ultimately boils down to needing things, whether it's your closet, your inbox, or your house, to be "just so." This can tie in with perfectionism, where you have to do something over and over again until it's exactly to your liking.

- **Contamination:** Perhaps the most well-known, this is when someone obsesses about getting sick and/or infecting others. This can look like intense fears of getting HIV/AIDS, of eating uncooked chicken that will give you food poisoning, or of infecting someone with a disease when you give them a hug, for example. Excessive cleaning, especially with washing of the hands (where they can become raw and bleeding), as well as avoidance of certain places (hospitals, restaurants, amusement parks, etc.) or people (kids and/or the elderly), are all common signs.

- **Scrupulosity/religiosity:** Rooted in one's morals, this is when you fear that you have sinned or wronged someone in a grave ethical violation. As a result, you may engage in compulsive praying as a way to relieve your guilt, or you may check in with cultural and religious leaders to confess and "check" on whether you've atoned for your behavior and/or thoughts.

- **Real events:** This is when you obsess about something in your past, ruminating on a conversation you had or an action you took. You might worry that you offended someone, that they will act out against you and you may be punished or embarrassed for what you did. An example of this could include sending a flirty text message to someone you're dating and fearing that they'll misinterpret what you said. As a result, you might check your phone excessively.

- **Pure O (Obsessive):** This can include any of the obsessive thoughts listed above; they just don't include any apparent compulsive behaviors (though counting, praying, and mentally checking are compulsive behaviors that may not manifest as physical actions). An example is frequent rumination, sometimes through a philosophical lens, where you may wonder what the meaning of life is, whether you're truly happy, or whether you're making the "right" decision.[33]

Did any of these resonate for you? I realize that reading this may be making you very uncomfortable. Many of these are taboo topics that are often unspeakable—but not unthinkable. That is why OCD is so upsetting. It's the brain handing us the most unwanted thoughts and images and uncontrollably splicing them over and over to a host who doesn't want them. This is exactly what was happening to Luís. Without his consent, his mind was doling out what he felt to be the most repulsive images and fears, and yet he couldn't stop it. Feeling so ashamed, Luís was at a loss. He shared that in his family, mental health concerns were rarely brought up. He worried that his family would not understand his experience. He also shared that they were not supportive if medication was a recommended treatment. So, for years, he had been privately battling the demons in his mind, feeling like he couldn't tell a soul.

While he was very hesitant to share, Luís disclosed that he identified with the harm-based, contamination, and real-events subsets of OCD. The next step was to understand his level of insight regarding his symptoms. Some clients have good or fair insight, where they're aware that they're experiencing obsessive thoughts and/or engaging in compulsive behaviors. They know that their compulsive behaviors are not directly impacting whether or not their fears come true, even though it can feel hard to stop. Other clients have poor insight, meaning they struggle to identify that their thoughts and behaviors are connected to an OCD diagnosis. These clients experience even greater distress because they ruminate, worrying, "What is wrong with me that I'm having these thoughts?" For example, they often believe it's only a matter of time until they do actually harm someone because the thoughts feel so powerful—even though they desperately do not want to cause harm. They also might desperately believe that they *have* to carry out their compulsive behaviors or their worst fears will, in fact, come to fruition.

With OCD, people beat themselves up to a mental pulp. They'll say to themselves, "I must be a terrible, awful, or gross person because I am actually thinking about this." What they don't realize is that they cannot control these thoughts. In fact, the more they try to *not* think about their obsessions, the more the mind lasers in on the distressing cognitive pattern. Sadly, this poor insight impacts about 21 to 36 percent of clients, with 4 percent having absent insight or delusional beliefs about their symptoms.[34] And unfortunately for Luís, he demonstrated poor insight about his symptoms—through no fault of his own. He had trouble understanding that he was actively experiencing OCD and instead believed that something was truly wrong with him. He thought he was broken. He doubted himself because he feared that his thoughts were true.

That's why learning about OCD—and educating ourselves—is so important. If we can recognize an OCD thought for what it is, rather than buy in, we can name the game so much faster. This means that while we cannot stop the obsessive thought from happening (as you'll remember, we can't control much of what the brain sends to the spam folder), we do get to choose what pile we put that mental mail in. For example, if you're having the obsessive thought that your partner doesn't love you and you need to look through their phone to make sure they're not cheating on you—this is where you have a choice. Instead of going all in on the obsessive thought and taking it as truth, you can instead say, "I'm *noticing* that I'm having the same obsessive thought about my partner cheating on me. That's my brain doing its OCD thing. I have a choice in how I respond. I choose to not go through his phone, even though that may feel uncomfortable for me."

What's at play here? It's that empowered acceptance again. You accept that you're having an obsessive thought. Your empowerment comes when you *choose* to not engage in the compulsive behavior. This is taking the out-of-control (the obsession) and responding with an in-control action. Sometimes we call this "opposite action," when you make an intentional choice to do the opposite of what the compulsive behavior wants you to do.[35]

I realize this is much easier said than done. When we feel anxious, our minds feel so out of control. We feel unhinged. What's cruel is that we think by engaging in compulsive behaviors, like washing our hands excessively or avoiding certain people, we will feel better. Momentarily, we do. That sweet wave of relief that washes over us when we check or seek affirmation is addicting. Yet it's what's ultimately making us feel worse. You may think that when you engage in compulsive behaviors you're giving yourself a buoy, but it's actually an anchor that's pulling you down deeper and deeper.

It's when we learn to sit with it—our thoughts, our feelings, and our bodies—that we can feel grounded again. This isn't meant to be comfy. No one wants to look at their obsessive thought straight on. But it's when we face it fully, rather than run away, that we see our fear and our pain for what it is. We learn that we can in fact live with it.

The fancy therapy term for this is what's called exposure and response prevention therapy, or ERP.[36] Considered a first-line intervention for OCD (and many other anxious presentations, such as social anxiety, panic disorder, and phobias, among others), ERP is all about helping us expose ourselves to what we fear and then not engaging in the compulsive behaviors that have previously, though temporarily, alleviated our distress. An example would be having the thought that you could be developing psychosis (a common one I see in folks who have family members with psychosis and/or mania) and then choosing *not* to google potential symptoms of psychosis onset for the third time today. Another example is confirming one time that you locked the door, instead of five times, when you're on your way to work.

If this sounds hard—it is. ERP can be very challenging, but it's one of the most effective modalities. Here's why: when you choose to sit with the discomfort of facing your obsessive thoughts, you learn that they no longer have to hold power over you. Over time, you start to see your compulsive behaviors are no longer necessary to make yourself feel better. Why? Because you're learning to trust yourself. Each time you *don't* check, wash, or put things in order, you see that time goes on and you survived. The world didn't fall apart. You are learning that you can live with the anxiety, even if the waters you're in feel chilly.

This is where I love to pull in some of the skills from dialectical behavior therapy, or DBT. Initially developed by Dr. Marsha Linehan for borderline personality disorder treatment, one of the core tenets of DBT includes "distress tolerance skills," where we learn how to get comfortable being uncomfortable.[37] Yep, it's as simple (and difficult) as it sounds. When we understand that we don't have to run away from our pain, we learn that the pain isn't often as bad as our brains have built it up to be. We start to see that getting our blood drawn when we have a needle phobia, letting down a friend when we have social anxiety, or, yes, even having a panic attack is survivable. They're not a good time, but we still can endure, as much as our anxiety would like us to believe otherwise.

This is something Luís really struggled with at first. He was afraid of letting go of his compulsive behaviors because he felt that they were keeping a protective layer over him. He worried that without his excessive handwashing, circling the block, and text-message checking, things really would fall apart. I told him we would take it slow.

If you're starting to do this work yourself, I suggest that you take it slow, too. That's why it's recommended to create an anxiety hierarchy as a game plan.[38] This is where you write out different exposures based on the intensity of your fear and gradually build your way up on a scale of 0 to 100 (with 100 being the most intense level of discomfort).

One of the ways that we gauge the intensity of the exposure is by utilizing what's called the Subjective Units of Distress Scale, or SUDS.[39] So for example, let's say that you have a fear of speaking in public. You would start small, like asking a seat partner a question or raising your hand in a small group. This might be a level 20 or 30 for you. From there, you would build up to sharing an idea in a larger room full of people before going on to give a speech to a group. This may be more like an SUD level of 70 or 80. The key is that you don't start your interventions by giving a speech to two hundred people. If the exposure is too intense, you'll likely have a negative experience that reinforces feeling incompetent. This then affirms that it really is as scary as you imagined. Instead, start small so that you can gradually build up your confidence. Over time, you repeat these exposures over and over until your SUDS level lowers. It doesn't mean that you'll ever hit a level 0, but you can certainly see your activation level go down.

Luís and I developed his anxiety hierarchy so that he could identify his list of exposures to help him gradually work his way up. I'll share his as an example (though altered to maintain confidentiality). Keep in mind that some exposures are imaginal, as they either can't be carried out in person or they shouldn't be.

Here's Luís's anxiety hierarchy (remember to not compare yourself, as we all have varying levels of fear for different circumstances).

LUÍS'S ANXIETY HIERARCHY:

0: Watching a movie, playing with his dog

10: Liking a friend's social media post

20: Spending time with his dad on the couch; not sanitizing groceries

30: Being in the car with his dad driving; hanging out with friends and going beyond small talk

40: Only showering once per day; being around his dad in the kitchen while Luís cooks (as he would have a knife in his hand)

50: Posting on social media about an opinion that others may disagree with and then not checking for at least an hour to see what other people's responses were

60: Not circling the block while driving to check whether he hit someone with his car; washing his hands one time instead of three times before cooking

70: Cooking with knives with his dad in the kitchen; not checking his phone to see whether he said something wrong

80: Only washing his hands once instead of four times after going to the bathroom; not checking with friends to see whether he made them upset

90: Initiating a disagreement with someone; not using hand sanitizer twenty times a day

100: Imagining what would happen if he did in fact murder his father; imagining his own death if he were to die from an infection that came from not washing his hands

As you can see, this list is highly personal. No two people's anxiety hierarchies look alike. And whether or not you have OCD, you can benefit from becoming more intentional about identifying your fears and then mapping out how to face them.

Let's create our own anxiety hierarchy. Use this as an opportunity to identify something that causes you to feel fearful and map out some interventions that would help you face that concern in a gradual way. This is all about jumping off the diving board, but we want to start small rather than going straight for the high dive.

WHAT ARE SOME FEAR(S) THAT YOU'RE STRUGGLING WITH CURRENTLY? WHAT ARE SOME INTERVENTIONS, GOING FROM A 0 SUDS SCORE ALL THE WAY UP TO 100, TO HELP YOU FACE THIS FEAR(S)?

0: _____

10: _____

20: _____

30: _____

40: _____

50: _____

60: _____

70: _____

80: _____

90: _____

100: _____

If this list you created feels overwhelming, I get it. That's why you want to start small and work your way up. I know this plan feels counterintuitive. Indeed, anytime you face an exposure, you likely will experience a wave of anxiety. Your heart may race, you could feel light-headed, and your sense of nervousness will probably escalate. This is when you may notice your SUDS level jump from a 20 to a 60. It's at this point when we feel the strongest pull to avoid the exposure, or to engage in a compulsive behavior to alleviate our distress. This is often done innocuously. We continue with these behaviors because they momentarily relieve anxiety.

The problem is that every time we do this dance of avoidance, checking, or any other compulsive behavior, the wave of our anxiety gets bigger and bigger until we feel like it's impossible to ride out the wave. Before long, we want to get out of the water entirely. We want to stay home, bail on our friends, and keep ourselves safe by eliminating as many triggers as possible. Before we know it, we're struggling with agoraphobia, where we can't leave our homes and our friends have given up on inviting us to hang out.

Thankfully, there's a way out. ERP therapy operates on the idea of habituation. Here's how it works: while the wave of your anxiety spikes when you first face a fear, anxiety levels ultimately go down when you tackle that fear over and over again. With each exposure we see that the wave's peak gets smaller. We begin to get desensitized to the threat. This works on a behavioral level. When we witness for ourselves that we can survive our anticipatory anxiety and our feared situations, the brain starts to believe that we just might be able to manage it. This is why it's so important that we show ourselves we can sit with the discomfort of our distress. It reminds us that we're often far more resilient than we realize.

I've done this work myself and I get what a delicate dance this is. That's why I highly recommend working with a provider who specializes in ERP to guide you through this process. I've seen how ERP can be life-changing and I've also seen how it can be traumatizing when it's not done well. After grappling for years with emetophobia, I decided to give ERP a try. Even though I knew it would be uncomfortable, I was sick (pun intended) of ruminating about getting food poisoning after meals, scanning the streets for vomit whenever we walked outside, and avoiding places such as bars because I could possibly see someone get sick. The biggest way that it was impacting me was that it was completely impeding my decision to think clearly about getting pregnant someday.

Now, I completely empathize if you're hesitant to start this kind of therapy—I know I was: "You mean I have to actively face my biggest fear? Yeah, I don't think so." But my distress was too great. You know if you've been there before (or if you're there right now) that you can reach a point where you're willing to get uncomfortable if it means relief could be on the other side. That's where I was when I decided to start ERP.

I worked with my own therapist to create my anxiety hierarchy. I started with things such as looking at pictures of vomit and cleaning Mochi's vomit. It got harder when we worked our way up to watching videos of people vomit. My therapist would sit alongside me in session as we watched people's ridiculous YouTube videos where they would drink dyed-blue milk and proceed to throw it up. Even though this work was challenging, I ultimately found that it was helpful. I was no longer checking the streets for vomit, and I could even watch movies where people threw up—though you still won't find me readily watching *The Sandlot* anytime soon (that carnival scene—IYKYK).

Eventually, as we worked our way up my anxiety hierarchy, my therapist thought it would be helpful for me to make myself vomit. I felt this was a questionable intervention. It seemed like it was bordering on self-harm to make myself sick, but I wanted to show that I was a "good" client. I learned a lot about my desire to please others through this process: I told her I was game for this challenge when in truth, I really wasn't—nor did I need to be.

We decided that I would take NyQuil (as it's often made me throw up in the past). I remember eating my dinner with a sense of dread, knowing that all too soon it might be looking back at me. I went to sleep groggy only to wake up in the middle of the night feeling nauseous and on edge. Ultimately, that night led to the worst panic attack of my life. I have never violently shaken, cried, or felt as if I were crawling out of my skin like that. My SUDS level was 100. It was way too much. All this, and I didn't even throw up! I learned a lot through that experience, but overcoming my fear of personally vomiting wasn't one of them. If anything, it only traumatized me more.

Going through this myself, I'm now exceptionally cautious when going through exposures with clients. Given that these fears are often deeply embedded, and can be rooted in past traumas, the client has to be in control throughout the process. The therapist-client bond needs to be rock solid so that clients can voice whether an intervention is too challenging or whether they feel uncomfortable. You need to go at a slow and steady pace. Your exposures should never inflict direct harm on yourself or others for the sake of facing a fear—and if you have a provider who is encouraging you to do this, it's time to speak up.

When you are working with a therapist, there is an inherent power differential. You trust your provider to work in your best interest. While I don't believe my therapist meant to induce harm, I'm also keenly aware as a client myself how easy it is to want to do what we're told in the name of a treatment plan. But hear this: it is always okay to say, "No, this exposure exercise is too difficult for me." Just voicing your boundaries is doing great work. You're facing the anxiety of people-pleasing when you stand up for yourself. Remember—you are in the driver's seat, and no one should ever force you to go at a pace that makes you feel unsafe or too uncomfortable.

That's why it was so crucial that Luís had full consent throughout the process. We had a safe word that he could use whenever the exercises got too difficult. I always wanted him to feel challenged so that he could feel a change, but I never wanted him to feel like he was drowning in anxiety during an exposure.

Once he had coping mechanisms in place, including breathing techniques and distress-tolerance skills, he was ready. At first, Luís did great with the tangible exercises. When he could behaviorally make a change, such as not washing his hands as often or not circling the block, he was able to take action in a way that felt empowering. Just as ERP predicts, we started to see his anxiety around these fears go down. As he saw that his worst fears didn't come true, he learned that his compulsive behaviors did not need to dominate his life.

However, where we hit a snag was with the obsessions themselves. Unlike with the compulsions, which can often be targeted behaviorally (you either do them or you don't—unless they are mental compulsions, such as counting or praying, which can be harder to control), Luís struggled to reevaluate the validity of his obsessions. Here's why:

BUT IT'S NOT THAT SIMPLE

When we're struggling with OCD, or any form of anxiety for that matter, we want something simple: *answers*. When it came to whether or not Luís's worst fears would come true, he desperately wanted these answers from me, and I couldn't give him those in good conscience. We often want to know, with full certainty, whether something is going to happen or not. We want to be sure whether we're going to get sick or not. "Tell me whether my partner is going to leave or stay." "Assure me that I'm going to get fired or that I'm not." I've seen the pleading eyes in many a client.

Of course, the honest answer to all of these questions is "I don't know."

I know that's the last thing you want to hear. It certainly was for Luís when he said, "What do you mean that you can't guarantee that I'm not going to hurt my father?!" I could see the anguish in his eyes.

Sitting with the uncertainty of life can be enough to fully unnerve us if we let it. Having to hold that in-between space rather than receiving a full "yes" or "no" can bring us to a halt. But even if someone makes us a promise, nothing is ever guaranteed. I could make a false promise to Luís, but ultimately it would only be enabling his anxiety to perpetuate. He'd also be internalizing that he needed me to be the judge of his future. This would only disempower him further if he learned that others, and not he himself, determined the choices that he made.

You can see how this plays out with OCD. Take for example how Luís was desperately afraid of getting sick. Now, was it possible that he could get listeriosis from a cantaloupe? Yes. In fact, 1,600 of us will get infected this year and 260 will die from it.[40] And yet when you consider that we have, at the time of this writing, 329.5 million people living in the United States, that means you have—get ready for it—a 0.00000486 percent chance of contracting this foodborne illness. Scary? Sure. Unlikely? Very.

With OCD, we think the odds are stacked against us. We struggle to weigh the logical probabilities. The *chance* of something "bad" happening feels shattering. It's that "maybe" that completely sidetracks us. It feels too hard to live in a world that doesn't operate completely on all-or-nothing principles. This is often why we engage in checking behaviors with others. We want someone to tell us they won't leave us. We need others to confirm that we didn't hit that bicyclist. We need to search WebMD just one more time. It's never-ending if we let our anxiety run amok in this way.

Friend, these are false assurances. You're only feeding the anxiety beast more when you're checking, avoiding, or seeking enabling from others. I know it's hard to sit with the uncertainty. It may be that "I don't know" is actually the best response we can hear and tell ourselves.

Why? As much as it may hurt to admit, *who the hell does actually know?* Accepting that we don't have all the answers—and that we don't *need* to have all the answers—can bring us out of the mental hellhole that we all get trapped in. This was a fundamental lesson that Luís was learning in our work together. Sometimes he would still buy into his obsessions of harming his dad, though.

This is where I gave him some tough love. "Luís, I want you to do two things moving forward. First, I want you to begin trusting yourself more. You are a capable man, and you are in control of your behaviors. You don't want to hurt your dad and though we can't prove it with one hundred percent certainty, there are no signs that you are going to hurt him. Second, I want you to name the OCD for what it is. These thoughts of harming your dad are not coming from an internal desire to harm him—it's the OCD playing with your brain. When you have these thoughts, I want you to name them as such. Declare them as OCD—not as you—and know that you do not need to buy into what your brain is serving you."

In his quiet way, I could see that he was taking in what I was saying. As I normalized the patterns of OCD, sharing that what he experienced has happened for many other folks, I could see that he was beginning to see that it was his brain, and not his true desires, that had been causing him pain. He learned that his shame and self-disgust were just manifestations of his OCD. When he discovered this was the pattern of OCD, and not a unique sickness within himself, he started to feel much less alone.

A NEW WAVE TO RIDE:
Do you find that you struggle with some all-or-nothing thinking? Do you crave concrete answers? What are some situations or questions in your life where you can begin accepting not always knowing what the "right" thing is?

YOU DON'T NEED TO HAVE ALL THE ANSWERS

With OCD, and so many forms of anxiety, we struggle with the in-between. But you don't need to box yourself into "right" or "wrong," "good" or "bad." Sometimes it's both. We call this concept dialectical thinking, where we hold a both/and, rather than an either/or, mentality.[41] In a nutshell, this perspective allows us to broaden our view, holding that we can think and feel in a multidimensional way rather than box our thoughts and feelings into singular categories. This is something Luís struggled with, as he felt that he couldn't share his opinions and trust that his friends would still love him, even if they disagreed.

With OCD or just about any form of anxiety, we'd love for life to be simple. However, even the "good" person does bad things sometimes and "bad" people can surprise us with their kindness. When we label others and ourselves, we're creating some impossible expectations for one another. Inevitably, no one can be "right" or "good" 100 percent of the time. And yet, if we have no middle place to land, we quickly devolve into being "bad" or "wrong" the second we slip up. That doesn't leave much wiggle room—so you better not mess up.

It's too much pressure.

And while this is distressing to the average person, when OCD and anxiety are at play, it's a whole other level of dysregulation. Because we see being "right" and "good" as safe harbors that will protect us in the world, we so desperately want to meet those marks. I know Luís certainly did. He tried with all of his might to never mess up. As a result, he became a shell of a person with no opinions, no likes or dislikes, and, dare I say, a muted personality that made it hard for others to connect with him at times.

One of the biggest areas of focus in therapy with Luís was helping him learn that he didn't need to be—and in fact it was impossible to be—a totally likable, flawless person. The truth is, we can never please everyone. People will have their opinions of you and as much as you may try, that's something you'll never be able to control.

Anxiety makes us want to believe that it just might be possible, though. If we're more agreeable next time, perhaps they'll be nicer to us. Conversely, if we don't always stand up for our beliefs, then people will think we're not doing enough. Before long we're in a mental rip current where we're desperately trying to swim every which way.

We've got to start making room for the both/and in our lives. We have to make it okay to disagree with our friends and still be able to hang out together, like Luís had to do. It needs to be all right to be Christian and queer, like it now is for Nikita. It's okay to appreciate the sanctity of a relationship and still call off an engagement, like Jacob did. We often feel that we need to check certain boxes and meet all the criteria in each category in order to belong. This isn't belonging—this is exclusion.

By giving ourselves permission to think critically and deeply about our feelings, values, and identities and how they intertwine, we're able to hold the complexity they deserve. In turn, we can also then make room for relationships with other people who may hold different perspectives. Differences of opinion do not have to be a "bad" or threatening thing—even though our anxiety may like us to think otherwise.

This path takes patience and courage. When we're ruled by our fear, we often avoid any potential disagreement or crucial conversation because it could be uncomfortable. We worry that we could make someone angry with us, even if we have the best intentions. We can fear that others will write us off if we don't do or say the exact "right" thing. For folks with anxiety, this can be a debilitating pressure. Indeed, this is what Luís was so afraid of—that overnight he would be x-ed out by friends and family if he offered up an opinion (even if it was about something as innocuous as a movie).

Here's the thing: We are all human. Each and every one of us. While it can be easy to point fingers and blame others when they mess up, we're no better than the rest. We all mess up. Yes, sometimes we need a metaphorical burn to learn our lesson, but we don't want to scorch one another so badly that there's no opportunity for regrowth. We're all broken. And we're all trying to figure out how we can be kinder, more loving, and more patient humans with one another each day (let's hope).

This is where I saw Luís make some of his greatest strides. He began testing out the both/and in his life and being okay with not always being perfect. What would happen if he told his friends that he didn't like a certain kind of music or that he didn't want to go to the restaurant that others recommended? To his surprise: the world kept turning. In fact, his friends told him that they loved getting to know what he thought. It turned out that his indifference was distancing him, not protecting him.

He even started to see this with his family. He shared with them his OCD diagnosis and we explained the biology of his symptoms. His family started to support him, including learning how to not enable him when he showed checking behavior. To be clear—his family was still hesitant about the treatment plan. For example, they were not pleased when Luís expressed his desire, and the clinical recommendation from his doctor, to take medication. However, having done the distress-tolerance work as well as the dialectical thinking practice, Luís was able to hold that his family did not need to agree with his medical decisions for him to move forward. He could still maintain meaningful relationships with them, even if they didn't like his decision to take an antidepressant (which is often prescribed for OCD). He valued their perspective *and* he valued what he needed to feel better.

I was proud to see how Luís grew through our work together. Better yet—I loved seeing him be proud of the progress that he made. His OCD didn't go away, but for the first time, he was learning how to live with it. The look of shame he held in the beginning transformed into a look of hope. As Luís saw, it can get better—and it started when he was willing to get comfortable being uncomfortable. Another client, Colleen, was about to do the same.

CHAPTER FIVE

WHAT'S BELOW THE SURFACE

WHAT'S IN MY WATER IS NOT THE SAME AS WHAT'S IN YOUR WATER

It's one thing to read a client's intake paperwork. It's a whole other thing to meet them face-to-face. When I first read Colleen's form, I could tell she was hurting. She met the usual criteria on the Beck Depression Inventory (BDI): lack of sleep, difficulty eating, feeling guilty about anything and everything. She also endorsed some passive suicidal ideation, having thoughts such as "It'd be easier if I weren't alive." She struggled with anxiety as well, noting that she desperately worried about her future and whether or not people liked her.

Seeing her in my office, though, was a whole different story. Identifying as a bisexual, cisgender, Taiwanese woman, she had long, dark hair that framed her face. She was polished in every sense of the word— her clothes, her nails, her shoes—and looked immaculate from head to toe. But it was when she glanced up that I could see the tears silently cascading down her cheeks.

Colleen had lived a storied life. She had been brought to the United States as a child from Taiwan, though she had no conscious memory of this move. Before long, her parents left her in her aunt's hands, as neither of them seemed to want the "obligation" of taking care of her. For years, Colleen had to bear the emotional and physical burdens of living under her aunt's roof. Because of the simple fact that she was born female, she was treated as lesser-than in her family. She was held up against her two older brothers, and while they would get to play video games and relax, Colleen did all the chores. When she didn't do things perfectly, her aunt would yell at her and hit her. She would call her "worthless" and a "mistake." Sometimes, her aunt would even lock her up in the basement, in the dark, for hours on end to punish her.

It broke my heart to hear that Colleen had lived in this torture for years. Colleen told me that she would dress herself up daily in a smile and would act like "everything was fine." Her aunt would hit her in places where people wouldn't see, so no one knew how she was abusing her.

Adding to the pain, she didn't have many friends. As a bisexual Taiwanese woman, she told me that people at school would often bully her. In her words, growing up in a mostly Chinese community, she didn't feel accepted by her peers—especially given the history between Taiwan and mainland China. One of her strengths, though, as she got older was that she marched to the beat of her own drum. She didn't shape-shift to meet other people's expectations of her. She wore bold clothes. She spoke her mind. When she didn't fit the "traditional" mold of wanting to only date men, her peers excluded her even more. This hurt her deeply, but at the same time, she wasn't willing to forgo who she was to appease perceptions. This is one of the things that I loved the most about Colleen.

Even though she put on a brave face to the world, the years of abuse and exclusion made an impact. Colleen came to the conclusion that no one wanted her. Her aunt hated her femaleness (even though her aunt was a woman herself) and her parents were nowhere to be seen. Colleen felt utterly abandoned, and I could see why.

As a result of this pain, Colleen had begun cutting herself as a teenager. She told me that feeling the physical pain numbed the emotional pain. She had started to drink. Having sex with random people was another way that she would try to forget all of the hurt in her life. What Colleen was finding, though, is that the more she ran from herself, the more lost she felt. What began as an abandonment by others started to feel like an abandonment of herself.

Given that Colleen was desperately afraid of being left behind, had a series of unstable relationships, would act impulsively, felt chronically empty, and was also engaging in self-harming behavior, it became clear that she met criteria for borderline personality disorder (BPD). It showed up in our work together too, as she would vacillate between deeply engaging in the sessions and not showing up when she didn't feel like it. She was hard to predict. I believe this was part of her defense mechanism. When things got vulnerable, she would pull away if she felt like people got too close. She learned at a young age that she couldn't trust anyone, and sometimes, that included me.

While I hold transparency as one of my core values as a therapist, it's absolutely essential when working with a client like Colleen. I always wanted us to be on the same page and she needed to know that she was in the driver's seat. That being said, it's helpful for a client to know what kind of road we're on. That's why when it comes to BPD, which is unfortunately still stigmatized (and shouldn't be), I'm very intentional about how I communicate this diagnosis. In fact, much of the time, I'll actually bring out the *DSM-5* in session and go through the symptoms with my client so that we can collaborate to determine whether the diagnosis feels fitting.

I realize this may surprise you, and, sure, sometimes clients don't want to know a diagnosis, as they feel it gives them a label. I respect that. However, when it comes to BPD, we see that when folks are informed about their diagnosis, they have a clearer understanding of their symptoms and the treatment outcomes. In fact, one study found that when therapists did not disclose a BPD diagnosis to their clients, 100 percent of those clients left the treatment process.[42] Why? I would argue it's because, before clients even go to therapy, they can sense that something feels "off." Colleen had known for years that she felt "different" but couldn't understand why. Many clients, like Colleen, want answers and my belief is that when we have one, we should give it. It's a rupture of trust for a therapist to withhold something so meaningful as a BPD diagnosis. Knowledge is power. Teaching clients about BPD, including whether they meet diagnostic criteria, can turn the tide.

When Colleen learned that BPD is a lived experience shared by many (in fact, it's estimated that 1.4 percent of the population experiences BPD and almost 75 percent of them are women), she felt so much less alone.[43] As can often be helpful, I recommended that she join a support group for people living with BPD, and she was elated as she told me how there were other people who could connect to the intense emotions she felt. For the first time, she felt seen by others.

I wish I could tell you that Colleen's story is unique. It's not. Sadly, I'm sure that as you read this, you are thinking of the pains in your own life or what you've heard from close friends and family members. Even so, you may be wondering why I'm bringing up BPD in a book that is focused on anxiety. Here's why: anxiety, BPD, depression, PTSD, OCD, eating disorders—I could go on—so much of these disorders is fueled by *trauma*. The symptoms may manifest differently for each of us, but the underlying root is often centered in our individual and our collective heartaches. The pain of our past brings us to the pain in our present.

These pains can rock our worlds. They change us, and oftentimes not for the better. (Yes, post-traumatic growth is a thing that I'll cover in a moment, but wouldn't it be better if the trauma had never happened in the first place?)[44] Colleen should never have been abused by her aunt. It was and always will be inexcusable. And though not an unavoidable causation, in her case, that trauma likely contributed to the development of her BPD symptoms. While not a requirement by any means (many folks with BPD have *not* experienced trauma), it's not uncommon that people with BPD have in fact experienced trauma in their lifetimes. In fact, estimates from a range of studies show that 30 to 80 percent of folks with BPD have endured trauma at some point in their lives.[45]

Trauma can come in many different forms. The *DSM-5* defines a traumatic event as "exposure to threatened death, serious injury, or sexual violence"; it can be directly experienced or indirectly experienced by witnessing others, learning of something that happened to a loved one, or repeatedly facing aversive events (as in the case of emergency responders).[46] And even though about 70 percent of folks experience this definition of trauma at some point in their lives (with over 30 percent endorsing at least four or more traumatic events), it's not a given that a person will go on to develop BPD, PTSD, or another mental health condition for that matter.[47] There are so many factors at play, including our genes, our environment, and our lived experiences, that can impact whether or not we experience symptoms.

Trauma shows up differently depending on the circumstances. There's been a designation of "large-T" traumas and "small-T" traumas or "micro-traumas."[48,49] Large-T traumas can include singular events such as natural disasters, mass shootings, or car accidents that can impact communities, families, and individuals. Micro-traumas are the daily cuts that build up over time, including bullying and microaggressions, and lead to a lifetime of collective traumatic experiences. Furthermore, some of us experience complex trauma, where we're enduring frequent, large-T traumas, such as ongoing physical and sexual abuse, living in poverty, intimate partner violence, or being a victim of war or discrimination, among other examples.[50,51]

In Colleen's case, it was all too much, as she was experiencing complex trauma for years throughout her childhood. Enduring regular though unpredictable physical abuse, parents who left her, and unstable friendships was more than enough to contribute to her symptomatology. Time and time again, Colleen came to expect that others would be cruel to her, that the world was unsafe, and that she didn't belong.

WHY WE REALLY ARE GENERATION ANXIETY

The story of Colleen's trauma really didn't start with her, though. Inter-generational trauma is all too real, and we've got to talk more about it. Though I never met Colleen's aunt, I'd venture a strong guess that she has her own tales of trauma, as she had to leave her country in Tai-wan and start over in the United States. As Dr. Sandra Wilson writes, "Hurt people hurt people."[52] (Not that this is an excuse or that being hurt automatically means you will hurt others as a precursor.) Sadly, when this pain is unresolved, we can get hurt the most by the people we expect to love us the most. Colleen's aunt pushed her own pain onto her niece, from woman to girl, day after day.

And just as bad: our countries, in all their brokenness, can hurt people and families beyond measure for centuries. Even as policies on paper can change, those emotional and physical scars are inherited well beyond the bodies that originally received them. In the United States, when we look at our history and acknowledge the lasting impacts of slavery, stealing lands from Indigenous tribes, and placing Japanese Americans in internment camps, among so many other horrific exam-ples, there is no way that we can deny the intergenerational trauma that has been passed down—and how it still is impacting those living today. It's no wonder that the descendants of the people who survived these atrocities live in daily fear and are distrustful of law enforcement, our economic structure, and the government at large, not to mention that they are actively enduring their own present injustices. They have not been protected and in fact, they have intentionally been maligned. We cannot deny this reality and it's up to each of us to be a part of changing this.

These crimes can have extensive effects. Even though we may not have directly lived through the atrocities of our country's history, our bodies may say otherwise. We can be impacted on a biological, microscopic level. These inquiries into the effects of intergenerational trauma began when researchers started studying Holocaust survivors and noticed that, in some cases, the children of concentration camp survivors seemed to be more traumatized than the survivors themselves.[53] Since the 1990s, these studies have gone even further, examining the impact of generational trauma on gene expression, a field of study known as epigenetics. One significant study found that children may be affected by exposure to parental trauma not only before they were born, but before they were even conceived.[54] All this to say, our DNA can literally be modified because of the pain that our mothers and fathers, grandmothers and grandfathers, and generations prior endured.

We're more than our cells, though. These narratives of trauma are embedded just as deeply. Rightly so, many of us have learned from our families that the world is unsafe and that people cannot be trusted. As people have witnessed one horrific act of injustice after another, we would be foolish not to. And yet, interestingly, one study found that teaching children to fear the world, something that about 53 percent of parents do, correlated with less success, less job and life satisfaction, poorer health, more depression, increased suicide attempts, and "less flourishing."[55] Then again, it's a lot easier to tell your children that the world wishes you well when you've been in a place of power and privilege all of your life, as had family members in generations prior. When you don't have to fear the unexplainable and unpredictable hammers of life, you're much more *free* to "flourish."

Given this, it makes sense why we are collectively Generation Anxiety. Biologically, historically, and emotionally, anxiety has become etched in our coding. For many of us, it has been steeped in our tea that we are not protected. Indeed, so many of our parents and grandparents haven't been. Our families have fed us user guides to keep us hyperalert. It's been done with the best of intentions. And while we need to integrate this intergenerational *wisdom*, there's a part of me that wonders: What if it can be different with us?

Yes, we may be a generation marked by anxiety and depression right now. Some people mockingly call us "snowflakes" because of it. But the fact that we have the capacity to feel deeply shouldn't define us negatively—if anything, that capacity to care is a strength, not a weakness. Just as we hold pain in our blood, we also hold power, too. Contrary to how some may frame us, I believe we are much more than our fear. While we would never choose the situation we've been dealt, we can take what we've been given and make something better. After all, if our genes can be changed based on the traumas we've endured, can they not be changed by the positive strides toward healing that we take as well? Who said we can't be the comeback kids with the comeback genes?

Indeed, various studies are showing that change is possible. We are seeing how mindfulness, exercise, eating nutrient-dense foods, not using substances to excess (especially nicotine and alcohol), and reducing stress, among other tools, can all play a part in changing the script.[56] What we do to our bodies changes us on a cellular level. For example, practicing mindfulness can help reduce the size of the amygdala (that lovely fear center we've been learning about) while thickening the gray matter in the prefrontal cortex, which helps us plan, problem solve, and navigate our emotions.[57] Another example: changing your diet and refraining from inflammatory-inducing foods (here's looking at you, ultraprocessed foods) impacts our gut microbiome. When we put foods such as salmon, spinach, cauliflower, and strawberries in our bodies, they act as protective agents against depression.[58,59,60]

All of this was incredibly empowering for Colleen to learn. While she had before felt like she was predetermined to carry out the same harmful patterns as her aunt (indeed, about 30 percent of abused and neglected children go on to abuse their own children), she learned that she had the power to change the narrative.[61,62] It wasn't just something to hope for: there were steps she could take to create direct outcomes that broke the generational cycle of abuse.

In our work together, Colleen began practicing mindfulness on a regular basis to learn how to respond instead of react, especially when it came to refraining from impulsive behaviors. She integrated distress-tolerance skills as she began coping with her feelings rather than escaping them by cutting her arms. She developed a healthy sense of trust with others, learning how to let people in who earned her respect, rather than doing so solely because they gave her attention sexually. Colleen was changing her behaviors with intention, and slowly but surely, this was likely changing her biology in a biofeedback loop that was working for her in the best way.

More than anything, I don't want you to read this section of the book and believe that you are destined to be anxious. It's not fated. We are not doomed to live a life of panic and worry just because it's in our history. Our parents and the generations before them are *part* of our story. But they are not our entire story. Ultimately, you get to write this chapter. With the pen in your hand, it's your responsibility to show up intentionally. We do not need to succumb to the narrative that it's all just too much and that it's beyond our power. That's how systems of pain, trauma, and injustice perpetuate.

And yes, let's be real, these problems are bigger than you or I. They're bigger than our parents and their parents. We are living in a world that is built on generations of pain, where there have been winners and losers, takers and victims. For hundreds of years, wounds have been ignored. It hasn't been okay and it's still not okay.

If we're going to face our anxiety and heal this intergenerational trauma, it's got to be done on a collective level. Our systems—and our perspectives—need to change. We each can play our part in rebuilding these broken systems by helping more than ourselves.

When I say that anxiety can make us selfish, this is what I mean. Our worries can pull us in so deeply that all we can see is ourselves and our personal problems. Our empathy is shattered because it's shrouded by the cloud of a scarcity mindset. We think we don't have enough to keep ourselves safe so we rarely look out to see how we could help a neighbor. We keep ourselves small and as a result, our anxiety tends to worsen with time. Interestingly, it's when we are willing to expand

and put ourselves in someone else's shoes that we can finally help one another out. In the end, we all feel better because we've been a part of the solution rather than the problem. We can learn to look after one another rather than just ourselves.

This is where empowered acceptance comes back to the forefront. We have to acknowledge what has been broken . . . and then we need to do something about it. We can choose to make it better—both for our own safety and so that our intergenerational trauma doesn't continue to get passed down out of necessity. We'll know we're making progress when parents don't have to worry that this is the last time they'll see their kids when they drop them off at school. It's when people do not have to follow a different protocol because of their race if they get pulled over for a traffic stop. It will be when folks feel like they can wait for the subway safely, no matter how old they are, what language they speak, or what they look like. It will be when people like Colleen feel that they can ask for help when they're being abused. I know this all sounds idealistic. But I'm not giving up hope. It's when we've given up our hope that we have the opposite of empowered acceptance: apathy. I refuse to accept *that*.

USING YOUR PAIN FOR A PURPOSE

Our traumas, both those on the individual and collective levels, can change us. We've just noted how these wounds can live on—but it's a more complicated story than it seems. It's not always for the worse. While few of us would choose to have endured our pains, we do see that post-traumatic growth occurs for about half to two-thirds of people who experience trauma.[63] This can include an increased sense of gratitude for life, more meaning in our relationships, feeling emotionally stronger, a greater connection to values, and a more profound sense of spirituality.[64] Going through pain in our lives often causes us to see the world through a different lens. We may start to see the little moments as precious rather than as inconsequential.

This always makes me think back to gratitude and how healing it can be. Not to be taken as a token of toxic positivity, of "just looking on the bright side," gratitude is instead about broadening our perspective to once again hold the dialectic. Pain *and* joy, loss *and* gain—it can be held together. This perspective can ground us when we're lost in our pain. When our precious pet passes away and it feels traumatic for us, we can also hold that it has been a tremendous gift to know the unconditional love of an animal. When our partner or parent is sick and we worry about what will happen to them, we can hold how special it is that we care so deeply about someone in the first place. Gratitude is not always a given, but when it's there, let's sop it up—like a delicious piece of sourdough bread with some olive oil.

Engaging in a gratitude practice on a regular basis is restorative to our souls, especially to those of us who have experienced trauma. We know that gratitude helps us physically by lowering our blood pressure and improving our immune function, and it helps us emotionally by warding off depression and anxiety while improving our overall sense of well-being.[65] And because our brains are hardwired to skew negative, we have to fight that much harder for what is going well in our lives. That's why I like to have my clients practice what I call the "Five Daily Gratitudes," to help them stay aware of the good, rather than just focus on the negative. The more specific you can get, the better.

Don't just state what may be the obvious for you. When asked what we're thankful for, we tend to name low-hanging fruit. We say, "I'm thankful for my friends, my family, my health, and my home." Given that many people don't have these things, these are indeed things to be thankful for if you have them. But they're too broad and you know that you're "supposed" to say them. When we recite these things, we often don't experience that profound sense of gratitude somatically in the body. One way we can experience a deeper connection to gratitude is to get specific and center in.

This was something that I integrated into my work with Colleen. While we spent much of our time processing the trauma she endured, we also took our time to explore what was going *well* in her life. It wasn't about putting silver linings on her pain. Her trauma was her trauma—there was no pretty bow to put on top. But I also wanted Colleen to know that her trauma did not have to steal her future as it had robbed her past.

Once Colleen began integrating a sense of gratitude, we started to see a dramatic difference in how she lived. Rather than just going through the motions, she began noticing and eventually looking for things that made her smile or laugh each day—whether it was a child giggling next to her at the park or a beautiful piece of clothing she saw when she was window shopping. Her gratitude practice was mindfulness embodied and I saw it restore her. It wasn't that she was ignoring her pain—it was just that she was making more room for the good that she hadn't been seeing before.

Let's practice our own Daily Gratitudes. Try this out for a week and see whether you notice any shift in your mood. I'll share mine as an example. I happen to be in New York for a work trip today as I'm writing mine:

1. **Listening to Taylor Swift's "Welcome to New York":** Ever one for a good cliché, I loved the quintessential moment of riding in the taxi and just watching people walking by on a summer afternoon in Manhattan. If only I spotted Taylor herself.

2. **Hotel robes:** They instantly put me in a good mood and I *instantly* have to put one on.

3. **Meeting new people at a new restaurant:** After the pandemic, there's something about seeing people face-to-face, especially for the first time. It's almost like watching a movie and then seeing the actors in real life; 3-D has taken on a whole new dimension for me.

4. **Good books and bathtubs:** Bathtubs are my favorite place to get lost in a book.

5. **Nostalgia:** I'm on a heavy dose of it as I'm reminded of all the memories that I have from visiting my husband while he was

in law school. We were long-distance for three years while he lived here. I can remember those sweet times all over again and it makes New York feel even more magical.

I invite you to write your own Five Daily Gratitudes. Take five minutes to reflect on the moments when you caught yourself smiling today. Even if you are going through a painful time right now, you can use this as an opportunity to see the fireflies in your darkest of nights. Both can be there.

MY FIVE DAILY GRATITUDES:

DATE: _____

1. _____

2. _____

3. _____

4. _____

5. _____

HOW DO YOU FEEL AFTER GOING THROUGH THIS EXERCISE?

_____

_____

_____

_____

If you want to take it to the next level, share your gratitude with your friends and family. It has a profound effect. We are so impacted by the emotional states of others and when we share our joy with others, it's contagious. You can thank your mirror neurons in your brain for that. These brain cells respond equally when you are doing an action yourself and when you witness someone else doing an action.[66] It's why when we see someone crying, we often begin to cry ourselves. The same goes for gratitude—when we hear about or see someone's happiness, our brains feel those same effects internally. Your delight is my delight, and my delight can be yours. Perhaps even as you read my example, it brought a smile to your face. This is just another example of how we can collectively connect and heal when we share our happiness with others.

TO THE CHILD WITHIN

Even with the ideas of post-traumatic growth and gratitude, this chapter may be heavy for you. And while we may not care to admit it because we minimize our pain or it feels too hard to face, the trauma we experience, especially at a young age (as was the case for Colleen), can shape us. What's so hard about this particular pain is that it can feel invisible—even to ourselves. We often have no conscious memories of these wounds and yet they mark our bodies and brains nonetheless. I knew this to be true in my own life when I had to acknowledge how the trauma I went through as a child impacted me still as an adult.

You're familiar by now with how I've grappled with emetophobia throughout my life. It's tortured me in a variety of ways as I've grown up and yet, all throughout my childhood and even into early adulthood, I never knew *why*. It wasn't until I was in my psychodynamic class in graduate school that it dawned on me.

It was about my mom.

I know, I know. A common therapy trope. But in this case, it was true.

When I was about two years old, my mom was diagnosed with Stage 3 breast cancer. It turned out she had a lump in her breast before she got pregnant with me, but, even as a nurse, she was repeatedly told she was "crazy" for believing that at thirty-five years old, she could have breast cancer. Finally, after years of her seeing the lump grow, someone believed her.

What happened next were years of surgeries, including a mastec-
tomy, hair loss, chemotherapy, and, sure enough, vomiting. As I was a
toddler then, I remember none of it.

While my conscious memory fails, I'm told that my mom was *very*
sick. I know she tried to shield me from her pain. In fact, I was frequently physically removed from my house to keep me from seeing her
so sick.

As time marched on, I never pieced together how my mom's cancer
shaped how I showed up in the world. The trauma was so deep that I
couldn't see it—I could only feel it. When you feel something almost all
the time, you don't realize that it may not be "normal." Panic attacks,
anxiety around peers, and seeking an excess amount of control was just
part of my daily experience. I was unknowingly living a life of frequent
aftershocks when I couldn't remember what the actual earthquake
felt like.

And then that one day in class it hit me. It became so obvious, as it
only does after you've processed something. I realized that vomit represented everything I feared—a lack of control, something that makes
you different, something that pulls you away, and at worst, death. For
someone like me who tries (sometimes all too hard) to give off that
same polished presence as Colleen, getting sick is the antithesis of looking like you have it together. It's vulnerability in the flesh.

Getting sick meant that I could lose everything—that it could be
the beginning of the end. It meant that at two years old, I could lose my
mom. That I wouldn't even remember her if I had lost her then. The
little girl who was wounded with fear was still showing up as an adult
wrecked by daily bouts of anxiety.

Fast-forward thirty years. I'm so grateful to tell you that I didn't
lose my mom then and I still have her now. I'm beyond lucky that I even
get to write that sentence.

And yet—I carry those wounds with me and I feel them now.
Reflecting on our past and how it has brought us to our present isn't a
futile endeavor. In fact, one of the most meaningful exercises that I do

with many of my clients is having them write a letter to their younger selves. No matter how much we've grown up, we all have that little person inside of us still. That person reminds us of where we've been. That person remembers.

Given Colleen's history of generational trauma, I invited her to write her own letter to little Colleen—the one who would get trapped in the basement, sitting in the pitch-black dark in suffocating heat. This form of letter writing, often seen in narrative therapy, can be an incredibly healing tool.[67] When Colleen engaged in this exercise, it was one of the most powerful moments in our work together when she read that letter aloud for herself. It was an act of coming back to herself when she had felt that so many had abandoned her before. Even though some may say it's a little "woo-woo," writing or speaking to ourselves is an open act of acknowledgment. It's the antithesis of abandonment, as we come back to revisit our young selves. We are saying to ourselves: "I see you. I see what happened. I am here to love you now in the way you should have been loved at the time."

And now I invite you to write your own letter to your inner child. You may feel hesitant to put pen to paper, but I don't think it's by happenstance that you're reading this book. Don't stop yourself from writing because you're afraid of tears flowing or anger swelling. Let it bubble up to the surface for you and breathe into it. Set aside some time in a safe space to say what you wish your younger self could have heard at that time. If it feels hard to get started, here are some prompts to guide you through:

- When is a time in your life that you remember feeling scared, in pain, or confused?
- What do you wish you could have told your inner child in those moments when you were anxious or hurting?
- If you felt abandoned or life felt out of control, what do you wish could have been done differently? How would you make a choice now as an adult to protect that younger version of yourself?

If you feel inspired to continue healing your inner child, there are so many ways to get in touch with the younger self that still lives inside of us. Many of us cut ourselves off from that version of ourselves—we block off memories, things we loved at the time, and that childlike sense of curiosity and play because the vulnerability feels too great. While we can't change the past, we can begin having corrective experiences in a safe way where we learn to re-love what brought us joy or heal what brought us pain. What's different is that we can parent ourselves—this time in the way that we wish it would have been done. Unlike in childhood, where we have so little control much of the time (let's be honest—we're often at the mercy of the adults around us), as adults we have more power to choose the outcome and resolve our narrative.

Here are some ways to reconnect and restore your inner child:

- **Look back on pictures from your childhood.** Think about or write a message of healing to the child you see looking back at you. Frame it and put it up as a reminder of your dedication to taking care of that child within.

- **Join an intramural sport, take a dance class, or do another physical activity that you enjoyed as a child.** Get back into that state of play. Perhaps if that activity became excessively competitive or a source of pain, you can repair that relationship with a new experience of it, particularly without any parental or coaching pressure.

- **Do some artwork.** As children, many of us painted, drew, colored, or sculpted. Taking time to do some art is a way to express and process what happened in your childhood while also reflecting on how things have changed in the years following.

- **Do a mindfulness exercise to revisit your younger self.** Go back to a time in your life when you'd like to bring yourself a sense of healing. A warning: this can be a very powerful and emotional exercise, so you may want to do this with a therapist present.

- **Spend time and play with other children.** Whether it's babysitting, interacting with family members, or even just observing how children engage when you see them, notice their innocence, their curiosity, and their fragility. Give yourself compassion when you consider how you existed in the world like this at one point. If you find that you struggle with self-blame or inappropriate guilt, this can be a way to reconsider who was responsible for your well-being as a child. It was your caretakers' and not your responsibility to look after you.

LEARNING TO LOVE YOURSELF THROUGH IT ALL

When I first met Colleen, she was so hard on herself. One of my biggest goals for Colleen was that she would come away with a sense of self-compassion—not just for that little girl inside but also for the grown woman she was now. My hope was that she would learn that it was okay to be kind to herself—that she wouldn't fall apart even more if she allowed herself to be loved from within. So many of us believe we have to be hard on ourselves—even cruel—if we want to get anywhere in life. Whether we're like Colleen and we've internalized that individual harsh voice (in her case from her aunt), or we take this message from society at large, many of us are brutal to ourselves. We say to ourselves, "You're such an idiot!" or "I can't believe you said that. They're going to think you're so stupid." We have a false impression that these berating words are making us better.

Surprise: they're not. In fact, these callous ways that we are speaking to ourselves are making us sick, emotionally, mentally, and physically. Before we know it, these thoughts can become so automatic that they feel inherent to our core sense of self. We begin to feel helpless and hopeless that our situation can improve. Not only has this been shown to increase the likelihood of experiencing depression, it also amps up our perfectionism (which is not actually a good thing) while limiting our ability to both see and engage with opportunities that can benefit us.[68]

However, practicing self-compassion, something that may not come easy for many of us, yields a wealth of positive benefits. Simply put: self-compassion is when we give ourselves permission to be a friend to ourselves. This improves our overall mental health while increasing our sense of resilience.[69] It's one of the best things we can do and yet so many of us withhold it from ourselves.

It was hard for Colleen to tap into self-compassion, as she didn't even have a great friend or family member to set an example for how she should be treated. Worse yet, she feared that if she was kind to herself, she would *really* fall apart. She thought her internal meanness was the only thing holding her up. You too may worry that if you're compassionate with yourself, you'll become lazy, foolish, or incapable. Others may have made you believe this through the years.

Trust me, the wheels will not fall off the cart if you're kind to yourself. In fact, thousands of studies have shown that practicing self-compassion contributes to more fruitful relationships, *less* fear of failure, increased motivation to fix mistakes, and improved body image, among other benefits.[70] And if you're hesitant to try, practice self-compassion for a day. I realize it's a mindset shift that can feel insurmountable when you've been used to mentally beating yourself up for years. So instead, dip a toe. Try it on and see what happens. When you notice that your world doesn't fall apart as that cruel inner voice would like you to believe it will, you might want to be kinder to yourself on a long-term basis.

Let's practice this shift together. It's hard to reframe our thoughts if we don't know what they are to begin with. Start by identifying what your negative inner critic tells you. If you're having trouble homing in on it, listen for the bully in your brain that intimidates you, insults you, and makes you feel inadequate. Next, we'll practice shifting our response. This isn't necessarily about completely changing your mindset (which can feel impossible at first). Instead, it's about reframing your perspective to include a broader, more realistic approach that allows for possibility rather than certainty. Remember that while we can't control the inner critic that pops up automatically, we do get to decide how we respond to it. We can choose kindness to ourselves in these moments. Be the loving parent to yourself that you may have wished you had.

A NEW WAVE TO RIDE:

Do you find that you struggle with self-compassion? What are some ways that you can practice being kinder to yourself?

When the time came to end my work with Colleen as I was finishing my training, I felt a tremendous sense of gratitude that she and I got to travel alongside each other for a while. Goodbyes with clients are never easy. The more time that I've spent with a client, the harder it can feel. Given Colleen's history with abandonment, I was nervous that she would see this as another experience where she was being left behind.

I was so wrong. Colleen was okay—more than okay, in fact. She decided that she wanted to continue on with another therapist. She was ready to keep learning and healing herself, even if that meant building trust all over again with someone new. Even though I was leaving this part of her journey, she was no longer leaving herself.

Perhaps some people in your life may have come and gone recently. Maybe you've been the one who needed to swim into different waters. Sometimes we're meant to swim alongside each other for a short time, and other times, it's for a good long while. However long we're in each other's company, I think we can all learn from one another. While I hope I helped Colleen, I know she helped me just as much. She taught me the power of showing up for yourself when no one else will. She lived out how to love yourself and how to bravely be who you are. I can still hear her drum's beat to this day. She encouraged me to march to the beat of my own drum a little more confidently. Now that you've swum alongside Colleen, I hope you start marching to the beat of yours, too.

CHAPTER SIX

FOR WHEN YOU'RE IN SHARK-INFESTED WATERS

Jordan had a great laugh. He had a contagious energy. Just by being around him, you felt your own mood instantly improve. He was one of those people. I would quickly learn that this was both a strength and a defense mechanism for him. Standing over six feet tall, Jordan was a Black, atheist, gay, cisgender man. He had never been to therapy before, and he found his way to my office because he was a "little" stressed-out.

I can often tell with folks that they're in distress before they even start to speak. Like with Nikita or Mikaela, their eyes are filled with pain and their story follows suit. Some clients manage to unabashedly share the highs and lows of their life story in a fifty-minute intake.

This wasn't the case with Jordan. In fact, after a few sessions, I was wondering why he was in my office in the first place. He had no trouble filling me in about his life as an attorney, all the dating he was doing, and how he was settling into life in Los Angeles. Yes, he had a lot on his plate, but he was also a social butterfly who seemed to be flying along just fine. What was I missing?

Now, I'm all for building rapport and taking time to connect with a client (in fact, I would argue, and the research shows, that the therapeutic relationship is the most important aspect of treatment).[71] I never want to force a client to disclose something prematurely before they're ready. Weeks were starting to go by, though, and while I was now well versed in Jordan's social life and caseload, I had a sneaking suspicion that there was more to the story than Jordan was telling me. I knew that if I didn't say something, we could be spinning our wheels for months. And I've seen it enough to know that sometimes a beaming smile can be just as indicative of pain as the tears that readily flow. I had to say something.

Eventually I interrupted, "Jordan, may I ask you a question?"

"Of course. I tell you everything. What do you want to know?"

"I know we have our sessions each week and you tell me about all the comings and goings of your life. On the surface, everything seems to be going exceedingly well for you. And yet, I can't help but wonder if we're missing something . . . Am I missing something?"

Jordan's face fell flat. He wasn't laughing anymore. In fact, I'd never seen him get so quiet.

I waited in the silence—not wanting to rush him out of this moment.

Eventually he opened his mouth. "Well actually, there is something I haven't told you yet."

I continued to wait and just gave a simple head nod. In these moments, you never know what a client is about to say.

Quietly he said, "Last year I tried to kill myself."

The air was still. Both of us held our breath for a moment as we waited to see how the other would respond. As we sat in the space, Jordan started to silently cry.

I could see in that moment that those tears represented so much to him. He had held them in for so long. He was crying for the amount of pressure he felt—the need to always have it together. The pressure to be *perfect*. Crying for the unrealistic demands that were stacked on him on a daily basis that didn't seem to be going anywhere anytime soon. He was crying for the little boy who felt like he constantly had to please and exceed everyone's expectations. With each win, he regularly heard that he "surprised" people when he excelled.

In the silence, his tears were finally free to come out. The trappings of his smile could no longer hold in his pain.

When I saw Jordan sitting with his suffering, I thought about how strong he'd had to be for so long. And while it made me sad, it also pissed me off. The fact that this sweet man felt that he had to constantly entertain, inspire, and appease others, so much so that he attempted to take his own life, made it abundantly clear how much our society has become a relentless pressure cooker. With the endless monotony of milestones to accomplish, Jordan had met every mark and then some. But as time passed, he felt that it was never enough—and he felt like others were always expecting more. He shared with me that it was especially burdensome for him as a Black man to feel the weight of obligation not only for his own life, but for his community that he wanted to make proud. His biggest fear was letting people down.

While you may or may not resonate with Jordan's lived experience, there's a common theme here that brings many of us to our brink: we're people-pleasing in excess. So much of our anxiety is rooted in not wanting to disappoint others. We will burden ourselves as long as it will keep others comfortable. We've handed over our well-being because we want people to believe that we've got everything under control. And as much as it seems like we're destigmatizing mental health, perhaps the biggest lie is how much we act like we're fine when we're not. After all, therapy is helpful for others but not for us because we're doing great! (And all the while we're silently dying inside). Jordan was doing this on a daily basis. He would take on cases at his firm that he didn't have the capacity for. He would continue dating partners whom he wasn't really interested in. To the rest of the world, he was golden. Even in our therapy sessions, he would keep things light so that I wouldn't have to sit with the emotional labor of his pain.

When we live for the happiness of others, we lose ourselves in the process. Yes, there's something to be said for compromise and working with others to ensure a net positive outcome for all. But if we're so busy trying to pacify those around us, not only do we find ourselves in a state of burnout, we also lose all self-respect because we're unwilling to honor our boundaries. Before we go on, let's build more personal insight into this. Here's a list to help you recognize how many people-pleasing tendencies you may have.[72,73]

SIGNS OF PEOPLE-PLEASING:

1. _____ I feel like I need to say yes to every opportunity that comes my way.

2. _____ I often say "yes" quickly and then regret it immediately after.

3. _____ I have trouble confronting others when I'm upset or concerned.

4. _____ I pretend to agree when internally I really disagree with what's being said.

5. _____ I worry that if I make others mad, it will permanently burn a bridge.

6. _____ I'd rather feel overwhelmed than disappoint someone.

7. _____ I have a hard time breaking up with partners because I don't want to hurt their feelings.

8. _____ I'm friends with people whom I don't really enjoy being around because it's easier to go along with it than to end the friendship.

9. _____ I'm often the first person people turn to when they need help.

10. ____ Self-care and personal time tend to be last on my list.

What came up for you as you went through this list? Did anything surprise you? Like with perfectionism, we are often socialized to believe that people-pleasing behaviors are a *good* thing. We don't conceptualize them as harmful. We're told that if we're helpful, agreeable, and involved, we're upstanding citizens making the world a better place. If we say no, or we disagree, we're cold, selfish, and unfeeling people who lack compassion for others. You can see how this all-or-nothing thinking rears its ugly head once again as we separate people into the "good" and "bad" categories. To bring in the dialectic: you can be both kind and helpful while also not being available all the time.

You may be wondering how we got here. When we throw anxiety into the mix, especially when it's got a social flavor to it, we get this heaping serving of people-pleasing where we utterly lose ourselves in the process. Many clients like Jordan feel that they don't actually know who they are anymore. We've lost sight of what we're interested in, what our values are, and whom we want to have in our lives because we've been living to placate others for so long. We've sure as heck lost sight of our calendar, as it's filled with obligations to everyone else but ourselves. Free time runs low and resentment builds high, but we just keep trucking along because we love feeling like we've helped in some way.

This pattern gets reinforced with time, too. Why? Because most of us love a people-pleaser. We'll drive an hour to get lunch with you so that you don't have to leave your house. We'll talk to you on the phone at two in the morning when you're stressed, and we don't say boo when you never call to ask how we're doing. We're the first to help you set up your party and the last to leave to help you clean up while you're passed out on the couch. A people-pleaser is a damn good friend, and you probably don't even realize it.

And that's the thing—you likely don't even notice that your friend is struggling with people-pleasing because they make life look so easy. They may seem blissfully happy. They are your friend who laughs at all your jokes and makes you feel adored, and you've probably never had a fight with them. If I were to ask you to describe them, you'd say they're just the "nicest person alive." That's probably how many people would describe Jordan.

Exceptionally hard truth, though? Sometimes they are the friend who *isn't* alive anymore. They are the friend who felt like they could never share how much they were hurting. They are the friend who was willing to forgo their own happiness for yours. They are the friend who was in so much pain but was so busy hiding it, they may not have even fully known it themselves. These are the friends who complete what seem like surprise suicides because we had "no idea" how much they were suffering . . . until it was too late.

I'm grateful every day that Jordan is not one of these statistics. The fact that he is still alive is not lost on me. And I know as you're reading this, you very likely are thinking of someone you know whose death or suicide attempt was an utter shock to you. In fact, 50 percent of us know someone closely who has died by suicide. This is understandable, given that we lose someone every eleven minutes in the United States to suicide.[74,75] It adds another layer, though, when there were seemingly no signs. It makes us question everything when that friend or family member—the one who appeared to have it all together—is no longer here with us because of their own doing.

That's why I want you to go through this chapter knowing where you stand. If you identify as a people-pleaser, my hope is that you can recognize the signs that you're being taken advantage of, while learning how to advocate for yourself. And if you're not in the doormat camp, I want you to learn how to support those who struggle with people-pleasing so that you do not unknowingly perpetuate cycles of over-stepped boundaries.

KNOWING THE SHARKS IN YOUR WATERS

It's hard to know how to protect yourself, though, if you don't know what you're defending yourself against. Many of us are in shark-infested waters and we don't even know it. Because we are socialized to sacrifice our own bandwidth to help others, we're often surprised and worried when we find our mental health is in the gutter as a by-product. We get confused, asking ourselves: "If I'm taking on this team lead at work (even though I'm not getting promoted or a pay raise), shouldn't I feel grateful because I'm making a positive impact and they see my potential? Why do I feel so exhausted and angry?" Or we doubt ourselves by saying: "If I'm being a good friend, staying up multiple nights a week to help my best friend process her breakup, why am I feeling so resentful? What's wrong with me that I'm not a better friend? I should be glad that she feels like she can turn to me. She clearly needs me."

Red alert. If you're falling under the assumption that you're not a good friend when you're already bending over backward, or that you're "lucky" to get all this extra work without the change in title and compensation, we've got to talk. Not only are you in shark-infested waters, I fear you've put on a seal costume, my friend. Worse yet, if your friends, your partner, or your boss makes you believe that you're *still* not doing enough when you're doing everything you can, we're now officially in the shark cage, just waiting for the bars to break. We've got to find a way out.

It's hard to know how to respond, though, if you're not aware of what kinds of sharks you're dealing with. All we know is that we feel awful. Many of us have been living in anxious need of approval for so long that we think it's normal to have overbooked calendars, no sleep, and a searing resentment underneath our incessant head nodding. Isn't that just what everybody does? Yeah, not so much.

Let's then break down the various sharks in our waters. As we do, I want you to be mindful of what sharks seem most prominent for you.[76]

1. **Our own minds:** We are often our own worst predators. We attack ourselves with cruel words that leave us internally shaking. We say to ourselves that we're "stupid," that "no one likes us," and that we don't "deserve" to find joy in life. We call ourselves a "failure." Things like imposter syndrome (which is not an official diagnosis, by the way), where we feel like we don't deserve to be in certain spaces or at a certain level, can really

flare here as we scare ourselves into believing it's "only a matter of time" until people find out "who we really are."

2. **Society at large:** As saddening and maddening as it is to say, there are still so many collective sharks that haunt us individually and systemically. We see racism, sexism, homophobia, and ageism on a regular basis. Every day, people are victims of religious persecution, as well as discrimination because of their national origin, ability status, parental status, or socioeconomic standing. This isn't even an exhaustive list. And while we can sometimes see these sharks a mile away, what makes them even scarier is that they can camouflage like no other. They can be right in front of us, and we still can miss them. Whether it's because we've been swimming around them for so long or because there are just so many of them, we have to get better at identifying these sharks and naming them for what they are. After that, we've got to give them a good punch to the gills so these fear tactics change. There's simply no place for these sharks in our waters. While I have a great deal of respect for actual sharks, these metaphorical sharks need to go extinct.

3. **Other people:** Yep, we're going there. Some people in our lives are sharks, whether they are bullies IRL or little internet trolls who dwell in caves. These sharks kill the mood and make us feel like we need to constantly watch our backs. And while this is frustrating, it can be just as taxing, if not more so, when the sharks are our very own family members, friends, and coworkers. These are people in our lives who should help us laugh and find joy. It's extra painful when the people whom we want to get vulnerable with are the ones who terrorize us, shame us, and make us doubt ourselves. Even more confusing, sometimes our loved ones can be compassionate, only to turn on us when we least expect it. No one is by any means perfect, but it's hard when the care we get from our closest is based on contingencies or when it's rooted in unpredictability.

A NEW WAVE TO RIDE:
As you read through this list, which sharks feel most relevant in your waters? How do you see these people and/or experiences causing you distress in your life? Furthermore, how are you responding to these sharks? Are you setting boundaries and swimming away or are you chumming up the waters and waiting for trouble?

Jordan was struggling with all kinds of sharks in his waters. He was internally so harsh on himself and bullied himself on a daily basis. He constantly put pressure on himself to be the best. He felt guilty if he allowed himself to rest. He was afraid of what would happen if he slowed down, and over time, his self-worth became rooted in his successes rather than his innate being. Part of our work was helping Jordan realize that he didn't need an impressive résumé to be a worthy human being. This was hard to parse, though, as Jordan's accomplishments made him feel somewhat protected from the sharks of racism and homophobia. He told me that as a gay, Black man, he felt that his achievements could buffer him from the pain of systemic barriers. He felt that if he became a partner, bought the dream house, and drove the nice car, people might leave him alone. And while so much of therapy can include challenging faulty thinking patterns, who was I to contradict this belief? We both knew that there may have been a sick truth to it. This is another example of why "just think differently" is a false narrative. Yes, we can shift perspective, but Jordan's perception of his reality was unfortunately accurate.

Before I met him, this pressure to "prove people wrong" became too much for him. As we explored why his suicide attempt happened, he told me that the constant obligation to be everything to everyone was unsustainable. He didn't see how he could keep on living like that for another forty years. He was already worn-out at twenty-eight.

It didn't help that some of the sharks in his waters were sometimes his own parents. While entirely well-meaning, they wanted *so much* for their son. Throughout his entire life, there was a constant pressure to be the best. Whether it was playing on his high school basketball team or moving across the country to go to a top law school, they cheered for Jordan each time he was at the top of the charts. He felt so loved in those moments, he would tell me. When he wasn't winning, though, or when he decided to take a break, his parents would get deafeningly quiet. Though they were not openly disapproving, their silent side-eyes made Jordan feel like he was letting them down the second he exhaled. That's how he learned at a young age that rest was for the "lazy." While it was unspoken, he wanted to make all of the sacrifices his parents made worth it. He saw how hard they worked with multiple jobs, rarely complaining. He appreciated everything they had done for him. One of his greatest fears was appearing ungrateful for everything he had been given. That's how he ended up taking on more and more—and doing so with a smile on his face. By his midtwenties, though, it was so much more than he could hold, and he broke down.

My heart ached for Jordan. While on the surface we had very little in common, I resonated with the crushing weight he felt to always do more. Maybe you can relate, too—even if you have little in common with Jordan or me. That's the thing—even though we all may have different demographics and different lived experiences, that mechanism of anxiety that propels us to push ourselves constantly can be a shared experience.

I'll never claim to know exactly how Jordan felt, but I do know that I can empathize with his experience. My own therapist expressed a similar concern for me when she reflected on my own people-pleasing tendencies. I should have known that I struggled with overdoing it when my tagline in high school and college was "I may not be the smartest, but I work the hardest." I remember my dad vehemently praising me for this phrase. Looking back, I now see how problematic it may have been.

I was telling myself two powerful and unhelpful statements when I would proudly repeat this harmful mantra. One, I was saying that I wasn't bright. I felt that I didn't have what it took with my intelligence alone, so I needed other tools to buffer it. As I see happen for so many young women, I felt like I had to at least work the hardest at making myself as attractive as possible to earn a seat at the table. (I'm not making this up either—the halo effect where we perceive attractive people as smarter is unfortunately a real thing.)[77] Because of this pressure, I would never go out in public without makeup on, and I was dieting on Weight Watchers before I graduated high school. It was all I could think about—how much I weighed, what people thought of my gummy smile, and how I measured up to others. It was exhausting to feel like I was never "good enough." I saw how unsustainable this way of living was because I was more unhappy and anxious than ever.

I got sick of living this way. I realized that obsessing over a smaller pant size wasn't worth sacrificing my happiness any longer. I started eating what I wanted again, and I went out in public more and more without a caked-on face. I realized that if other people judged me for my appearance, that was a projection of their own insecurity.

Even so, as I get older, I still struggle sometimes with feeling like I need to be "put together" for people to listen to me. I told myself that I could at least work myself into oblivion to meet my goals. The equation was simple: meet your goals and *then* you can be happy. If you "make it," then you can finally have a right to love yourself and receive love from others. A winning strategy, really.

Relentlessly, I said yes to every opportunity that came my way. I lived and breathed by my to-do list. Each feather in the cap helped me keep at bay the thought that I wasn't worthy on my own. Before long, I was deep down the rabbit hole of hustle culture and didn't see anything wrong with it. And I was praised adamantly for it.

"How do you do it?" "What's your secret?" "I want to know your time-management skills!"

Oh, my secret? Just a deep-seated insecurity that I'm nothing without my résumé, title, or track record.

There's another "secret" that needs to be named as well: I've had the privilege of *having* the time to pursue my goals. I'm vehemently aware that many do not have the time or resources to go after their deepest dreams and are just trying to survive paycheck to paycheck. Time is one of the most lucrative currencies and without it, many of us struggle to get ahead.

That's why when people say celebrities have the same twenty-four hours in the day, it's a total bogus claim. Sure, we all logically have the same twenty-four hours in a day, but most of us don't have cooks to make us healthy meals, assistants to take care of extra tasks, and trainers to help us exercise in our personal gyms. Many of us do not have this privilege of time, and how much we get can vary throughout our lives. I know that I have been fortunate to be gifted with time, even though my anxious brain has tried to trample it. I want to make that awareness abundantly clear as I share my experience. It's not just that I've earned things in life because I'm a hard worker—I've been granted the time to work hard on the things I'm passionate about in the first place.

With this at the forefront, I've learned that I no longer need to fall for the belief that I'm not smart and that I need to work hard to earn love. I don't have to buy into these myths that I'm lazy if I rest and I'm worthless if I'm not accomplished. Neither is true. These are lessons I'm reminding myself of every day. I'm teaching myself that I am intelligent and that my value is not based in my looks or what I do. I'm also learning that I don't have to constantly perform to feel loved. Maybe you can resonate with this—feeling like you're only as good as your recent Instagram post. What I'm finding, though, is that a life of obscurity is just as meaningful and beautiful as a life that is more forward-facing. Neither is necessary to find contentment in life. We are more than the number of followers, likes, and reshares that we get. An algorithm does not need to determine how we feel about ourselves.

IT'S ALL ABOUT WINNING THE SURFING COMPETITION

I doubt I'm alone in struggling with this. I could see Jordan feeling in his own way the weight of expectations himself, although his looked different from mine. I see so many of my clients grappling with this same externalized sense of self-worth. We feel like we need to get into the best schools, date the best potential partners, and get the best job if people are going to give us the time of day—let alone if we are going to give ourselves permission to be happy. With parents who cheered for us proudly when we were winning, we learned at a young age to equate joy and love with advancement.

And we wonder why we are Generation Anxiety. We've internalized that we can never stop. There's a sense of hungry desperation that makes us feel like we need to be everywhere at all times. We've ultimately made ourselves sick with exhaustion, and the only way we're going to get better is if we actually allow ourselves to listen to our bodies and change this cycle of endless pursuit. As a wise supervisor once told me, we need to move from human doings to human *beings*.

That's hard to do, though, when our generation has thrived on checked boxes. We have believed that if we hit our daily quota, *then* we will feel content. Jordan had fallen for this trap, thinking that if he did a little more, then he would finally feel at peace. Instead, our anxiety only fuels our endless list-making and calendaring. Before long, we're working on our birthdays and we haven't taken a vacation in two years. Jordan couldn't even remember the last time he had fun for himself.

And while part of our problem is trying to please others, we've also been trying to please ourselves. We feel that we can keep our anxiety at bay if we push ourselves from sunup to sundown. Many of our parents taught us this as well. We learned that if we played three sports, took AP classes, and got a promotion at a prestigious company, we were "good." If we didn't have multiple hobbies, took non-honors classes, and worked for a business that wasn't name-drop–worthy, we were "bad." We were *behind*. This usually wasn't said out loud, but these were the messages that many of us absorbed.

Full disclosure—I don't think our parents did this with malicious intentions. They wanted the best for us. Like coaches, they wanted to watch us win because they thought this would set us up for success in life. In fact, they probably thought it would alleviate our anxiety if we were winning in all things. Who knew that it could actually have a detrimental effect? In this way, we've learned that we're only as good as our latest achievements. Without them, we can feel like we are nothing.

If we're going to tap into less of an achievement-driven culture, we're going to need to forgo our people-pleasing tendencies. This begs the question: What would it look like if you stopped living for the approval of your boss, your parents, or yourself? Are you willing to find out? Your constant striving no longer needs to starve you of your sanity. It's okay to say no.

This was one of the major goals that I worked on with Jordan. As I'm keen to give clients homework, I encouraged him to take time outside of our sessions and take stock of how he was living his life. I wanted him to evaluate how his self-care was going and begin seriously taking some time for himself. Being the A-plus student that he was, getting the outside motivation from me to treat himself finally took hold. He was able to see that when he set boundaries, his world expanded in a whole new way as he finally prioritized what was most important to him. Not only did he get back into basketball (this time just for fun), he took himself on a trip to Jamaica and got a puppy. Instead of being first in and last to leave the office, he started working from home sometimes. He began exercising a few times a week, rather than billing for another hour. He had dinner with his parents more often, rather than calling for a fifteen-minute check-in every two weeks. He told them what was actually going on in his life, rather than just sharing his victory lap.

His priorities shifted. He began using his time differently and when people asked him for favors, he was more mindful about what he agreed to. He was exhaling. I saw fully how things had changed when I heard him laugh one day and it didn't sound like there was anything underneath it. His laugh could be sincere because he was finally allowing himself to cry, smile, be angry, feel scared—it was *all* allowed.

WHEN YOU DO HAVE THE POWER TO SET BOUNDARIES

And while some of us don't always have the luxury of setting boundaries in our lives, it's okay to exert them compassionately when we can. In particular, if you struggle with people-pleasing, this is where you can embrace the discomfort of respecting yourself. Take a moment to sit with that. There's a sad truth sitting there: **When we people-please, it is because we respect others more than we respect ourselves.** We come second. We think we're being selfish when we stick up for ourselves.

Now, why is this? People-pleasing is ultimately a form of avoidance. In this case, we want to avoid the possibility of anger and disappointment from others. We worry that we will permanently burn bridges if we stand up for ourselves. Our anxiety keeps us in check as the good little accommodators that we are. And that's the thing—our people-pleasing has been reinforced from day one. People love when we do exactly as we're told and applaud our willingness to always show up.

So why would you stop? It feels so good to get the pat on the back. Before long, we internalize that we are *needed*. Problematically, we also have learned that the best way to earn love is to give relentlessly to others. We fear that people will reject us if we show up simply as ourselves, without all the accoutrement of our favors.

Once we realize that this cycle has become toxic—you know, the one where people abuse all your energy and your resentment cup overfloweth but you just can't stop—it feels too late. We worry that if we were to make a change and speak up for ourselves, the world would spin on its head. People would surely leave us. We would be all alone. Abandoned. What good is a doormat after all if there is no one to walk on it?

I won't lie to you. When you do start standing up for yourself, some of the people in your life are not going to like it. They've been used to a relationship where you have been all the things to them—taxi driver, therapist, chef (likely all for free). When you start demanding respect, saying no sometimes, or expecting something in return, some people are going to start leaving some pretty nasty Yelp reviews because you raised your menu price.

And that's okay. You will survive.

When you set boundaries, you will see pretty quickly who loves you for who you are and who loves you for what you do for them. People will either honor the respect you're requesting or they will shame you for it. This gives you invaluable data, my friend.

Many of us are afraid of getting data that we don't want. We'll keep ourselves in a place of purgatory for months or years because we're afraid of people showing us their true colors. Boundaries can show how the people who seemed to love you may have only loved how you made them feel. Don't be afraid of finding out that truth. You don't need to keep swimming in shark-infested waters.

If you're feeling scared to swim into unknown territory—the kind where you actually push back against the sharks in your life—you're not alone. Jordan was petrified of setting limits with others. He was afraid he would get fired if he didn't work every weekend. He thought no one would want to date him if he wasn't always willing to drive an hour in LA traffic every week. But when I asked him if the way he was living his life was working for him, he replied tersely, "No." When I asked him whether he was willing to see what would happen when he did what he wanted, rather than what everyone else wanted, he cautiously said, "I guess I could try it."

We came up with a list for Jordan to practice. He communicated more clearly with his colleagues about his availability, rather than placing himself constantly on call. He told his dating partners that he couldn't drive out sometimes, but he was happy to have them visit him. While he was nervous about how these experiments would turn out, he quickly saw results. He learned who respected his time at work and they built stronger relationships. For the ones who didn't value his time, he eventually found new cases with partners who honored his schedule. Soon enough, Jordan had free weekends to enjoy as he pleased. He also learned that some of the men he dated seemed to be with him only when he was willing to brave the traffic. However, he also was able to find a man who was happy to compromise and drive out to him as well. Had he not set that boundary, he could have floundered in even more aimless relationships. Because he stood up for himself, Jordan found a man who adored him and whom he adored. The best part was that they could actually spend time together, because Jordan was learning how to set boundaries not just at home, but at work as well.

A NEW WAVE TO RIDE:

What are some boundaries that you can begin setting in your life? How can you stay committed to these boundaries, even when others may give you pushback?

HOW TO SWIM IN THIS NEW WATER

How do we actually set boundaries to protect ourselves, though? We're right back at that diving board where we're looking down into the abyss. It's scary to take the jump. When you've lived a life of people-pleasing, you usually know the outcome. People will be happy with you, while you will (semi) hate yourself as a result. The idea of telling people no or saying we're not available is pretty unpredictable—it's vulnerability at a level 10.

I want you to come back to the dialectic, though: you can both have boundaries and connect with others. You can still be an amazing friend and have time for yourself. You can be a loving child to your parents and still not live out every dream they have for you. All these things can coexist. It does not have to be one or the other. In fact, I would argue that operating on either end of the spectrum doesn't put us in a place of health.

I love the framework that John and Linda Friel present in their book, *Adult Children: The Secrets of Dysfunctional Families.*[78] They write about the three different kinds of boundaries that we can set, and as I describe each, I invite you to consider where you land:

1. **Diffuse:** For my people-pleasers, this is when you're too flexible with your boundaries and you say yes to everything and everyone. You feel overwhelmed and perhaps internally angry but struggle to stand up for yourself. You may feel like everyone is walking all over you, but your anxiety can block you from changing the behavior.

2. **Rigid:** The opposite of diffuse, you're quick to say no and you keep others at a distance. You don't trust others and you may struggle to connect because you believe people may be trying to take advantage of you. You have time for yourself, but you may also lack close relationships.

3. **Flexible:** The ideal way to hold boundaries, you can discern when to say yes and when to say no. You're in tune with your values, so you gladly commit to the opportunities and people who bring you joy. In the same vein, you're not afraid to say no when time doesn't permit or you're not interested. Because you respect yourself, you're also able to appropriately respect others by being honest about what you actually do and do not want to do. Lastly, you're willing to compromise, knowing that sometimes you can have your way and sometimes you can't—both can be okay.

If you find yourself in the diffuse or rigid category, consider being open to the possibility of responding differently. Our responses aren't fated. Our approach and our relationships are not going to change unless we're willing to do something about it. We have to actually take action and follow through. Changing your mindset isn't enough. Why? It's because our brains are so freaking smart. Simply telling ourselves that our worst fears won't come true if we stick up for ourselves only does so much. You have to actually show yourself that it can be different. Prove to yourself that you survived saying no to a "quick favor" or that you handled someone being angry with you if you turned them down. Here are some ways you can implement this if you struggle with boundary setting:

For those with diffuse boundaries:

1. **Slow yourself down:** Whether you give yourself a rule of waiting twenty-four hours before you give an answer or you simply start saying "Let me get back to you on that," give yourself a stopgap in responding. With people-pleasing, we have a knee-jerk reaction to say yes without really considering how the new obligation would fit into our lives. Slow. It. Down.

2. **Let go of external flattery to determine your self-worth:** Compliments are our weakness—especially when they're attached to a request. Because we associate being needed with being liked, we're quick to take the bait, even if it will put us out. Before you commit, ask yourself whether you actually want to take on this responsibility or you're just basking in the glow of validation.

3. **Practice saying no:** Just try it on. Whether it's a friend asking to go to dinner and you're absolutely exhausted or you've been asked to sign up for an extra shift at work, see how it feels in your body to say no. You likely will feel restless and guilty at first. Give yourself a day, though, to pay attention to any waves of relief that follow. You may be surprised by how good it feels to stick up for yourself. Also, the world likely didn't end as you may have imagined it would.

For those with rigid boundaries:

1. **Give people the benefit of the doubt:** When we're closed off, it's often because we don't trust people and we assume they're trying to hurt us. Instead, consider a different perspective that people may be wanting to help instead of harm you. Open yourself up to the possibility that something good could come out of saying yes.

2. **Embrace discomfort:** We often say no because we don't want to experience any pain. And while we don't need to make ourselves suffer, some of the biggest growth happens when we're willing to get a little uncomfy, whether it's trying a new workout class or tackling a tough project at work. Step into the vulnerability of discomfort and watch how you change for the better.

3. **Ask yourself the regret question:** Sometimes we can jump to an immediate no without asking ourselves whether we would regret never opening this new door. While you may be quick to turn down a date or decline that invite, is there the slightest chance you would regret not finding out what's on the other side? If so, then perhaps you take a peek.

Signs of healthy boundary setting:

1. **Asking a friend for perspective:** You're not afraid to seek counsel with others because you're aware that you don't have all the answers. You're willing to admit when you could be wrong, and you can integrate alternative perspectives while you come to your own conclusions.

2. **You're connected to your values:** You are going to have a lot of choices coming at you. It can feel hard to know what to say yes to and what to turn down. By centering in on your values, you're grounded in an intentional future based on what matters the most to you. Remember, values induction over pain reduction. You know that people will live through the disappointment of you turning down their offer. You don't sacrifice your well-being for someone else's satisfaction.

3. **You're willing to compromise and change your mind:** Never static, you're able to accommodate changes as they come up. You can admit when you're wrong, whether you've taken on too much and need to step back or you've been too firm and need to give a little more.

So much of the time we struggle with boundary setting because we have a scarcity mindset. We worry this will be our "last chance" or it's our only shot at a "big break," so we feel like we have to take every opportunity that comes our way. While we do want to challenge ourselves to keep growing, we don't want to squeeze ourselves into a pulp. When we're living in a mentality where our worth is defined by what we do, rather than who we are, our lives become a bucket with a hole in it—it's never enough. We constantly need more and more to feel like we have any value.

I realize this is one of the hardest nuts to crack. We've grown up in a society where we judge others by where they went to school, how many followers they have, and what kind of car they drive. We haven't been taught to find value in quiet afternoons, long conversations that don't have agendas, and walks where our steps aren't tracked. But it's okay to sit back and float in your waters. You can still have a productive and fruitful life that is rooted in times of guiltless rest. That is a choice you get to make. Maybe it's time to enjoy the water rather than feel like you always have to swim from one destination to the next.

Watching Jordan float back and enjoy the water around him made me feel so happy for him. The man I first met was inundated with the pressures of his life—he was living for everyone else but himself. The man I finished therapy with was still working incredibly hard—*and* he was taking time to enjoy his life at the same time. He had learned how to embrace the both/and, and he was giving himself full permission to marinate in what brought him joy. Don't forget that you can do the same.

CHAPTER SEVEN

KNOW WHO YOUR LIFEGUARDS ARE AND WHERE THEY ARE

Sometimes it's a parent who reaches out to me instead of the actual client. It's not uncommon that I'll get worried voice mails from moms and dads, asking whether I can see their child (a grown adult) as soon as possible. I'm always happy to oblige a consultation, but I go in a little more cautiously when this is the case. While sometimes we need a loved one's support to take that first step, I'm mindful of how much the parent wants the help for their child, rather than the client wanting the help for themselves.

I met my client Casey in this way. She was a straight, biracial (half white, half Latinx), cisgender woman. At twenty-six, she was in her first year of medical school and lived with two roommates. I met with her after her mom, Jessica, had disclosed to me what had been going on recently.

I learned that the harried call from Mom was after one night on Casey's recent spring break. Thinking that Casey was exceling in all things—she was in med school, had a loving boyfriend, and *seemed* happy—Jessica's world turned upside down when her daughter had a breakdown, sharing that she had been "hating" how her body looked and couldn't believe how "ugly" she was. Casey told her mom, "It's all that I can think about." Jessica couldn't believe it and was stunned to see how distressed her daughter was. Hence the phone call to me.

I see this pattern happen often with anxious folks—especially those with perfectionism. (I'm also all too familiar because I've done this dance myself.) Ninety-eight percent of the time, we have our ish together. We're collected, capable, and seemingly at ease. And then, get us in the right setting, and we can have a Category 5 meltdown of disastrous proportions. There's crying, there's yelling, there's utter bemoaning. Our loved ones are typically aghast at this juxtaposition and proceed to panic. They tell us we should get some support. We momentarily accept because we're in so much pain. The walls are down. This usually lasts for a night.

But then, by morning, we've magically collected ourselves. We're back to our painted-on masks and it's like nothing ever happened. The walls of the castle are back up.

When our loved ones say, "How are you doing after last night?" we respond with, "Oh, that? I don't even know what you're talking about. I was just tired." It was just a blip. Nothing to worry about.

So, when Casey came to me with nonchalance, I knew her own walls had been drawn back up. But thanks to her mom, the cat was out of the bag.

Casey had never done therapy before, which didn't surprise me. From her perspective, she had everything under control. Her mom had just caught her in a moment of weakness (that I was now privy to). And while her mom was trying to look out for her and get her help, it was going to be an uphill battle, as Casey was unconvinced that therapy would help. After all, we'd be exploring her feelings—something that she was disinclined to do unless under the most desperate circumstances. And yet, here she was.

When I'm getting to know a client, I always want to know the underlying reason why they're distressed and what motivates their behavior. Some would say Casey was a textbook type A personality. Highly achievement oriented, she went straight from undergrad to medical school and told me that she hoped to become the top of her class. While her drive helped her perform in many ways, this same drive also applied to how she ate. What began as a desire to eat "healthy" quickly devolved into orthorexia, where she would become greatly distressed if she was unable to eat "clean" food.[79] Before long, she would find herself obsessing in front of the mirror for hours when she ate the "bad foods" she "shouldn't" be eating. I referred her to a nutritionist to help with her eating patterns, and I focused on the body dysmorphia (which is in the same section as OCD in the *DSM-5*, by the way) so that Casey could practice accepting her body as it was.

Before we started with any interventions, I shared with Casey my conceptualization after we completed her intake. There were three key things happening, according to my assessment. First, as we often see for those struggling with anxiety, she had a deep need for control. Whether it was her grades, her appearance, or the food she ate—she wanted everything to be managed just so. Paying attention to how her body looked was a regular fixture in her day. She obsessed about how her skin looked and how her clothes fit. She cared more about what others thought when they saw her walking to class than how she felt in her own skin. She was emotionally cut off from herself. She shared with me that she rarely processed or even identified how she felt because feelings seemed out of control for her. She feared that, like a volcano, she might explode emotionally, so she kept her feelings locked down for as long as she could. She never cried if she could help it (and hence why her mom was so shocked that fateful spring break night).

Second, Casey had a deep insecurity within herself. Though attractive, she was always worried about how people perceived her. Fearing that she wasn't trendy enough or skinny enough, she felt that she would never be included by her peers. Even though she had so much going for her as a talented physician in training, her self-worth was rooted entirely in her physicality. When I said to her one day, "What if your appearance is actually the least interesting thing about you?" she replied, "If only." For Casey, it didn't matter how smart she was. She was only as good as her pant size.

Last, Casey did not know or trust herself. When I asked what she liked or what she thought, she struggled to give me answers. Wearing Lululemon every day, she told me that she had a hard time picking out what to wear because she was so afraid of being different. Judgment from others was her worst fear. I soon discovered where this lack of self-assurance came from as she would give me little clues.

"I can't decide how to do my makeup today. I'm going to have my friends do it for me."

"I don't know what I should eat this week. I'm going to have my boyfriend send over a list of groceries I should buy."

"I'm not sure what I should specialize in at med school. I'm going to see what my mom thinks I would be good at."

All said so innocently. In fact, Casey thought she was helping herself by asking for hourly input. As we would discuss in our work together, though, there's a difference between accessing resources and unconsciously seeking enabling from others to ameliorate our anxiety. When the latter is happening, as it was for Casey, it's an indication that our anxiety is controlling us. We are telling ourselves that we are not equipped to make choices on our own. By handing over our decision-making power to others, we are subversively saying that we are not capable of taking our own steps—and that we do not have the resilience to manage the outcomes. We'd rather put our fate in someone else's hands so that we do not have to take responsibility. So even though Casey tried to control her life as much as she could, it soon became clear how out of control she really felt. She was scared—and she needed everyone else to pave the way for her.

When we're unsure, many of us do the same checking behavior and we don't even realize it. We see nothing wrong with leaning on our loved ones. In fact, as we just covered in the chapter on people-pleasing, some of our friends and family *love* that feeling of being needed by us. It makes them feel special. And while there's nothing wrong with getting opinions or advice, we want to be mindful when we are taking their feedback as gospel truth. When we are letting the input of others determine our path, rather than making our choices from our own best judgment, we are telling ourselves that we don't trust our internal compass. We are saying that it's safer to rely on someone else than ourselves. That's a powerful message to tell yourself.

Where is that message typically coming from? Your frenemy: anxiety. Anxiety is telling you that your judgment is inadequate. It's saying that you'd be a fool to rely on yourself. And once you've listened to this voice long enough, you unknowingly hand over your self-confidence. Quickly growing out of control, your insecurity spreads and you need more and more external validation to move ahead. As for Casey, she was in deep and could barely recognize herself anymore. She was living more for who others thought she should be, rather than what she wanted for herself. But by the time I saw her, she no longer knew what she wanted in the first place.

KNOW WHERE YOUR LIFEGUARD SITS

Don't get me wrong: we all need people in our lives who support us. However, we want to be mindful of where the lifeguards in our lives are sitting on our beaches. Are your loved ones looking out for you on the shore, cheering you on and letting you know whether they see some sharks swimming nearby? Or are they on a Jet Ski with you sitting on the back, directing every which way you go in your water? You may not realize it at first, but your life is going to continue to feel half-baked if you are always allowing everyone else but you to call the shots. I know it can feel so good in the moment to have someone else take ownership of the outcomes of your decisions. Each time you do this, though, you're depriving yourself of your own strength. Before long, you'll feel too weak to swim on your own.

I think it's helpful to note some of these signs of enabling behavior because they're often happening without our realizing it. As we go through this, I want you to be mindful of how you may be asking others to accommodate you, or how you may have been appeasing others without realizing it. I also offer a way to refrain from enabling, which ultimately breaks this cycle of anxious checking behavior.

WHEN YOU'RE SEEKING ENABLING	WHEN YOU'RE THE ENABLER	A DIFFERENT APPROACH
You worry that things won't be okay, so you ask your best friend whether everything is going to be all right.	You don't actually know whether things will turn out okay, but you make a false promise to your friend and tell them it will all work out just fine.	"I don't know what is going to happen, but I do know that we will find a way to work through it."
You're scared that you're going to get sick, so you ask your mom if you could be catching a bug.	You have no idea whether they are going to get sick but you want to help them feel better, so you lie and say they won't become ill.	"I don't know if you'll get sick. Let's talk about how we would handle it if you did get sick."
You don't know whether you locked the door when you left the house, even though you checked it when you left. You plead with your friend to turn around so that you can check it one more time.	You turn back around after driving ten minutes and check that the door is locked.	You don't go back to check if possible. You reply, "Do you remember locking the door?" Encourage your friend to trust themselves and talk through how they can cope with their fears without engaging in checking behaviors.

You're not sure whether you should end your relationship with your partner, so you ask your best friend what to do.	Based on your assessment, you tell your friend whether or not they should break up with their partner.	Unless you're concerned about potential abuse, you ask your friend questions to help them come to their own conclusions.
You tell your roommate that you feel stressed-out.	You bring your roommate a bottle of wine to help them forget about their feelings.	You sit with your roommate over a meal and talk about what's been worrying them lately.
You feel self-conscious in your body, and you worry your outfit doesn't look good on you. You check with your friend to ask whether it looks like you gained weight.	You promise your friend that they look amazing and tell them it doesn't look like they've gained any weight at all.	You tell your friend that their weight doesn't define their worth. You might help them pick out a different outfit but at the end of the day, it's about owning the body you're in. You remind them that confidence isn't contingent on appearance.

When we enable others, it's often done from a place of love. We hate to see our friends and family struggling with anxiety. We want to help them feel better. In fact, for many of us, it feels cruel to not give in to the checking behavior. It's much easier to say "It'll be fine" when our best friend is scared about her dad's cancer diagnosis. It's much harder to express in truth, "I don't know what is going to happen, but I hope you know that I'm here for you."

We also often respond with false-hope maxims because telling an anxious person what they don't want to hear is anxiety-provoking in itself. We want to keep things comfortable. Being honest about the fact that bad things can happen can create some tidal waves. We don't always want to ride those waves ourselves. People may get angry or frustrated if we can't promise their safety. It's a lot easier to go with the flow and respond with an empty assurance. The waters temporarily calm when you say, "Nothing bad is going to happen. Don't worry." Little do you realize, it starts to get annoying when you have to give this consolation over and over again when your initial bout of enabling wasn't enough. Spoiler alert: it never is.

I was seeing this pattern play out with Casey and her boyfriend. She clung desperately to him because he steadied her nerves—or so she thought. Because she felt that she needed him so much, she would frequently worry whether he, we'll call him Seth, "really" loved her.

She would often ask him throughout the day, "Do you love me?" and "Are you going to break up with me?"

Initially, Seth typically responded with "Of course I love you!" and "I'm never going to break up with you."

While these answers temporarily relieved Casey's anxiety, the cycle didn't change—it was only reinforced. Casey was checking more and more, now multiple times a day. Before long, Seth was getting fed up with the frequent questions. What's worse, Casey was never feeling fully satisfied and she started to stalk his social media. Yep, she went there.

This was where I came in. I helped Casey name the cycle. She was feeling anxious and wanted affirmation from Seth. The more she checked with him, the more uncertain she felt. While Seth would tell her what she wanted to hear, it was harder and harder for her to believe him. Why? Because she couldn't *prove* that he loved her, and she couldn't be *certain* that he wouldn't break up with her. It was a classic case of anxious attachment. Something had to give.

I invited Casey and Seth to start responding differently. I encouraged Casey to refrain from asking these hot-air questions that she couldn't get answers to. I invited Seth to a session with Casey and coached him on how to respond when Casey was seeking validation. Rather than telling her what she wanted to hear, he learned to instead respond with

"Casey, you know how I feel about you. I'm not going to answer that question because we know it will actually reinforce your anxiety."

I shared with Casey that the validation she had been seeking was not going to satiate her in the relationship—it was chipping away at the relationship. Instead, she needed to see with time and through Seth's actions that he did in fact love her. She had to practice trusting him. She also needed to accept a hard truth: they may break up someday— and that would be okay. "Always" and "never" are two words that can't be promised in any relationship (even with marriage), as life is inevitably changing day by day. Even with the best of intentions, nothing is guaranteed. A hard pill to swallow, I know.

Now, remember how I told you Casey had trouble expressing emotion? Yeah, after we had these sessions, not so much anymore. The volcano erupted. When I shared these recommended changes in behavior, she got *mad*. Red cheeks, big eyes, shaking hands—she was hot lava. I had just thrown her world upside down by not guaranteeing that this relationship would last forever.

Casey jolted. "So, you're telling me that I should stop asking my boyfriend if he loves me or not?"

"Yep."

"And you're telling me that he's supposed to respond by saying that I already know how he feels, and he will let me know if he changes his mind?"

"Yep." I paused. "Do you believe that your boyfriend loves you?"

"Well . . . yes."

"How do you know?"

"He's there for me. We have so much fun together. The sex is great. He's my best friend, really."

"And do you trust that if he did want to end the relationship, he would do so in a respectful way?"

"I think so."

I waited a beat. "And let's be honest. Let's say your worst fear came true and he did end the relationship. What would you do?"

She admitted, "I would be really sad at first. Heartbroken, in fact. But I would also be okay. After all, I don't want to be with someone who doesn't want to be with me."

"So you're saying you would get through it?"

"I guess I would."

This was a big ask: not only was I inviting her to stop the behavior that she found so (temporarily) self-soothing, I was also prompting her support network to engage with her in a whole new way. I wasn't doing this to be malicious. I wanted her to see that she was much more capable than she realized. I needed her to know that she could handle pain and uncertainty—both of which are inevitable in life. Even though she didn't believe me at first, I wanted her to hold that she could be okay, even if she didn't have her lifeguard buoying her up.

Something powerful happened after this interaction. Casey decided to start swimming on her own. Before long, she began doing her own makeup, picking out her own clothes, and making her own meals—all without the input of the people around her. This may seem trivial to someone who doesn't struggle with this particular evolution of anxiety, but it was a big deal for her. She wasn't calling friends and family multiple times a day, asking for their input. It wasn't just the daily changes, either. After assessing her own values and interests, she chose to pursue obstetrics and gynecology, instead of relying on what her mom recommended from afar.

As she came into her own, it didn't mean that she wasn't welcoming of support. It's just that she wasn't relying on it to function. She told me that her relationships started to improve because the dynamic was shifting. It was less about asking for help and more about simply being together. There was no longer the inequality of the "helper" and the "helped." Whether it was with her boyfriend, her mom, or her roommates, Casey was showing up on the same level, rather than begging on her knees for what she should do with her day (or low-key, her life). She was standing on her own two feet.

The next problem, though, was that Casey didn't like her feet. Or her stomach. Or her face. Or anything about how she looked, really.

WE ARE GENERATION ANXIETY BECAUSE WE ARE GENERATION APPEARANCE

It's not by happenstance that Casey was struggling with how she looked. She had been primed to feel insecure. Especially regarding how she physically looked, she had internalized at a young age, as many of us do, that her worth was connected to how others viewed her. Perhaps you can resonate with this as well. In fact, it was crucial for me to include a chapter on the intersection of our appearance with our anxiety because I am seeing such an epidemic of body insecurity and unhealthy eating patterns. Other clinicians have shared with me that they are noticing more and more clients struggle with hating how they look. The research supports this too, as we are seeing increased rates of eating disorders and body dysmorphia emerge as screen time, social media, and filtered images have taken the world by storm.[80]

People aren't wrong about how much importance our society places on physical appearance. We have a real issue with body-size discrimination and we need to do something about it. There are entire books written about this and indeed, I recommend reading about the intersection between anxiety and appearance in greater detail. Our work in this domain is just getting started. We continue to need systemic change, where we notice our biases and we step in to stop them. The solution is not shape-shifting ourselves to win people over. The answer is not starving ourselves, exercising to excess, or making ourselves vomit (which actually doesn't make you lose weight in the long term, FYI).[81] Although our generation continues to be plagued by filters and an ever-increasing pressure to look like Barbie and Ken dolls, we can push back.

Our lives depend on it. When we starve ourselves or make ourselves sick to meet some unobtainable ideal, there are consequences.

Eating disorders are the second-most-deadly mental health concern after the opioid crisis.[82] In fact, we lose someone to an eating disorder every fifty-two minutes.[83] Many folks aren't getting the support they need, either. BIPOC folks are half as likely to be diagnosed or get treatment for an eating disorder, and they are significantly less likely to even be asked by a doctor whether they have any symptoms.[84] LGBTQIA+ folks are impacted as well—in fact, gay men are seven times more likely to binge eat and twelve times more likely to purge, while transgender college students demonstrate disordered eating at four times the rate compared to their cisgender peers.[85,86] And before we go assuming that people suffering from eating disorders look a certain way, it should be known that fewer than 6 percent of people with an eating disorder are medically diagnosed as "underweight."[87,88] Eating disorders and body dysmorphia can impact anyone, and it's bound up with our anxiety. In fact, 71 percent of those struggling with an eating disorder have another diagnosis. What tops the chart with a 53 percent rate of comorbidity? Anxiety.[89]

Our generation has sadly learned that striving for attractiveness is a false antidote to this anxiety and a way to wield power. Young women especially, who may feel like they lack power in terms of their knowledge, experience, or sheer personhood, have been taught that their looks can give them social clout. This has pitted women against women. We compare ourselves constantly to one another to know where we stand in the social hierarchy. We use our looks as a benchmark to determine whether we should feel confident or insecure. In fact, clients frequently tell me that one of the first things they'll do is scan a room to see where they fall in the looks lineup. Appearance has become an achievement in its own right. This is a lesson that we need to unlearn.

Now, to be fair, we have started to see some changes in the way that beauty is defined. The Westernized ideal of a woman being thin and tall, having light/tan skin, long hair, big breasts, large eyes, a small nose, and high cheekbones is changing.[90] Brands such as Fenty and Aerie have changed the game, especially since the days of Victoria's Secret and Abercrombie & Fitch, when many Millennials were finding their way alongside size 00 models and way too much cologne. Body mass index, or BMI, is no longer recommended as a way to define someone's health, as it didn't use representative data from the start (collected samples from white Europeans informed its categories).[91] We now know that the one-size-fits-all approach is outdated. We're also learning that weight doesn't necessarily correlate with overall body health. Smaller-size bodies can still have cardiometabolic abnormalities, while there is a prevalence of heavier-bodied people who are considered metabolically healthy.[92]

Still—we have a long way to go. Weight bias remains stuck on the scale. Many of us grew up with parents who told us that gaining weight was to be avoided at all costs. We were side-eyed if we ate a burger *and* fries. We learned in school that we were "unhealthy" if we had larger bodies. To this day, we continue to blame and shame people for their weight, believing they are lazy, unsuccessful, and not intelligent, among other harmful stereotypes.[93] Unlike with some things that we cannot change, such as ethnicity and age, we believe that people are irresponsible if they do not have a smaller frame. This may be a part of why we actually see higher rates of weight discrimination on an institutional level and interpersonal level, as compared to discrimination based on gender or race.[94] We think it's justified to discriminate based on someone's appearance because we falsely believe it's something we can control. And as our classic framework with anxiety goes—the more you try to control something, the more out of control you actually feel. It's no wonder our generation feels beyond anxious about our bodies. When we're told we "should" be able to contort how we look, and then we can't or it's not enough, we go into a tailspin.

This has led to an epic level of avoidance—where anxiety often leads us. We tell ourselves that we don't want to date anyone until we lose ten pounds. We don't want to go out with friends because we don't like how we look in our clothes or because we have acne on our faces. We don't want to have sex because we don't want to feel exposed in our bodies. At some point we have to say enough is enough. We can't keep letting society dictate the feeling that we don't deserve to date, go out, and have sex unless we look a certain way. At some point we have to step out and do what we want to do—no matter how we look. And if a person judges us or our bodies? That's on them. It's one thing to have personal preferences—it's another to shame someone who doesn't fit the stereotypical mold of beauty. Whatever that is. Each of us needs to define beauty in our own way. And then there's this: perhaps our beauty doesn't need to define us to begin with. There's so much more to us than just how we look.

OWNING YOUR WATERS

Like so many of us, Casey was avoiding so much of her life because she didn't like how she looked. She was paying the price. Because she was so deeply insecure, she would second-guess everything. She hesitated to wear color because it could make her stand out. She didn't want to raise her hand in class because people might judge her. She stressed about her food choices because they could impact how her body looked. Even though people make fun of the term "basic," she was aiming to be as textbook basic as possible. Why? Because she didn't want to be different. Being different could mean that she could be excluded or that people would think she was "weird." To her, there was no worse feeling. It was her primal trigger point.

Now, if a client wants to blend in because it suits them, I respect that. That's why I always assess how a client feels about their behavior. In Casey's situation, she shared with me that she would like to be more confident. She felt that she had been keeping herself boxed in but was too afraid to break out, and when a client lets me know that they want to feel more sure of themselves, that's my sign to activate empowered acceptance in our work together. Here's the process.

First, we have to acknowledge and accept what is. When it came to Casey, and for so many of my clients who struggle with their body image, we leaned into body neutrality work. Yep, you'll notice I didn't say "body positivity" here. While the body positivity movement began in 1969 with the fat acceptance movement, and undoubtedly continues to do some incredible work to this day, others have shared that the messaging "love my body" feels impossible to grasp.[95] While I still believe it can be a helpful framework for tying in self-compassion, I also get that the idea of unconditionally loving your body, though it sounds nice, can feel disingenuous.

That's why body neutrality—where you practice accepting your body for what it is and what it can do, rather than what it looks like—can be a more passable entry point, especially if you struggle with body dysmorphia and/or an eating disorder. I love how Anuschka Rees, author and body neutrality activist, describes this difference in perspective in her book *Beyond Beautiful*. She suggests that while body positivity hopes to change the definition of beauty in our society, body neutrality centers on changing the *value* of beauty of our society.[96] I find that incredibly powerful. Thinking about what it would be like to live in a world where our bodies could just be bodies and our worth isn't attached to how they look—it gives me goose bumps.

So that's where we started with Casey. Rather than encouraging her to practice disingenuous self-talk (e.g., "I love how my stomach looks!"), we instead integrated mindfulness to simply build awareness of her body and what it could do for her. An example of this included helping Casey acknowledge how her stomach helps her digest food so that she has enough energy to get through her day. By shifting this focus, Casey was even able to integrate a sense of gratitude for her body. It didn't mean that she loved how she looked, but she was beginning to understand that her body actually did a lot for her each day. Here again we're holding the dialectic of the both/and: you can both appreciate what your body can do and not love how it looks—and that's all okay.

I think it'd be helpful to lean into an exercise to practice for yourself some body neutrality. I invite you to list three parts of your body (perhaps name some parts of your body that you struggle to love at times) and note how those parts help you currently or have served you in the past.

PART OF YOUR BODY:	WHAT HAS THIS PART OF YOUR BODY DONE FOR YOU OR HOW DOES IT HELP YOU CURRENTLY?

How did that exercise feel for you? Did you notice any shift in perspective? If not, that's okay. Be patient with yourself in the process. If you've been hating on your body for years, it takes time to start viewing your body through a different lens. Perhaps a place to start is holding that it could be *possible* for you to accept your body as is.

I also began helping Casey detach her worth from her appearance—which was a journey that I was all too familiar with myself. Now, this is some of the hardest work that I have done with clients because, let me tell you, our beliefs about beauty in our society are *deeply* entrenched. Just as folks may have internalized homophobia, racism, and ableism, among other forms of discrimination, so many of us have internalized appearance bias. We shame ourselves for having wrinkles, cellulite, saggy skin, small breasts, big breasts, no butt, big hips, small muscles, acne—the list goes on and on and it's ever changing depending on what's trending. We hold a false promise with ourselves that if only we were "beautiful," then life would be easier.

In *The Beauty Myth*, Naomi Wolf breaks down how women have been socialized to obsess about our appearance to divert us from our rising power. Wolf shares how this impossible striving toward "flawless beauty" is an endeavor that leaves women bound up in self-consciousness and self-hate.[97] Though the book was published in 1990, it still rings true today. I was seeing it actively play out in how Casey talked about and saw herself.

For many of us, so much of our worrying is bound up with what we see in the mirror. And though we may not like to admit it, our appearance is not really something we can control. No matter how many diets, surgeries, injections, and creams are pushed onto us, there are many things about ourselves that are genetically inherent to who we are—our skin color, our cup size, our body fat percentage. There's only so much variability to what we're born with. We can fight against that, or we can accept (and not always love) the body that we see staring back at us.

Now, to be clear, if there are aspects about yourself that you want to change—I'm not going to hold you back if it makes you happy. However, I think we must ask ourselves *why* we're engaging in cosmetic procedures and spending thousands of dollars on body-altering processes. Is it because doing so makes us feel more confident? Are we aiming to please ourselves, or everyone else around us?

Some say go all in with the procedures, makeup, and hair coloring if it rocks your socks. Others are the polar opposite: don't shave your armpits, don't wear makeup, and flaunt your wrinkles proudly. If it makes you feel good and you're doing it for you—who are we to judge one another? It's when we're choosing for ourselves how we want to show up, and anxiety isn't dictating it, that we're winning the battle. This is the definition of empowerment.

So much of our distress around our bodies is rooted in our concern about how people will perceive them. But why should their opinions matter? Do these random strangers, or even the people closest to you, get to determine how you feel about yourself? If the answer is yes, I think we may need to reevaluate that one. When you have someone else deciding your self-worth based on their evaluation of your physical appearance, you are forgoing your power entirely. This is the opposite of empowered acceptance.

And let me ask a follow-up question here: Why don't *you* deserve that power?

Why aren't you enough on your own to decide how you feel about your body and how you live in it? I hope this book can be a jolt that gets you to realize that no one but you should determine how you feel in your skin. I realize there are larger systemic forces at play that make these mind games harder to win, but I will say this—the cycle starts to end when we stop buying into the myth that we need to look a certain way. It's simple and so dang hard at the same time. Be the way that you want to be. Unapologetically so. When you do this, your anxiety will likely abate. When you're not worrying about what everyone thinks (which you can't control anyway), your anxiety starts to lose its grip. The fear tactics of worrying how others perceive you no longer apply. You've got better things to do.

This is ultimately about giving yourself permission to own who you are—and it doesn't need to be contingent on how you look. This is the empowered piece—and it's where you need to take action. You can't think your way into being more confident. You have to show yourself.

One of my goals for Casey was to help her get more comfortable in her body. She often appeared very tight in session—her chest almost caved in on itself and her smile was fixed without showing her teeth. I could see that she was so afraid of looking like a fool that she constricted herself into nothingness. There was no goofiness—no element of play—in how she presented. Even across the screen, it seemed that it was hard for her to breathe.

I've seen this happen for many clients, where they've locked everything in place to prevent any potential misstep from happening. Avoiding embarrassment is their primary goal. When I see clients come in like this, it tells me that we need to loosen up. So what if your outfit looks silly? Or if you walk out of the bathroom and there's toilet paper on your shoes? The world keeps on spinning and you just proved your humanness. And believe it or not, when you're not perfect, people like you *more*. It's called the pratfall effect, and the idea is that people who are considered competent are actually more likable when they also demonstrate fallibility, whether it's falling down, dropping something, or flubbing.[98] Even if things don't go according to plan, people are connecting more to you when you show that you're just like the rest of us: imperfect.

So take your power back. Own your humanness. Embrace the weird. Once you realize that we're all our own brand of strange and embarrassing, you won't feel so singled out anymore. And remember— those who judge you have their own internalized pain that is getting projected onto you. Perfectionists often critique other perfectionists and it's because they view the world with the same harsh eye with which they view themselves. Once you break the cycle and realize that you don't need to live for that unhealthy gaze, you've set yourself free. Commence the happy dance—and please don't judge me for my moves.

A NEW WAVE TO RIDE:
Do you notice your appearance, and the potential judgment from others, impact your experience of anxiety? What steps can you take to practice embracing who you are, integrating both acceptance and empowerment with how you see yourself?

NO LONGER WEIGHT-ING TO FEEL BETTER

Casey came a long way in our work together, and I started to see her give herself permission to unwind from her tightly balled coil of anxiety.

However, as with all parts of the therapy process, sometimes the detangling gets too overwhelming. As I warned her, it takes time to develop the skills that come along with confidence building. It's a practice. I could see that she would get frustrated with herself if she felt that she wasn't making progress fast enough. I could also see her annoyance with me if I didn't help her improve at the pace she desired. When I didn't wave the magic wand that she wanted, she was disappointed.

Our patterns of growth are never linear. It comes with a slow and steady pace. Sometimes when anxiety is surging, we want our pain to be resolved once and for all. We get fed up when it doesn't work that way. Part of Casey's process was learning how to be patient with herself as she stepped into the person she wanted to become. She redefined her priorities. It was no longer about sculpting an exterior image so that people would hopefully love her. Instead, it was about deeply understanding the person underneath the hair, the makeup, the clothes. Just as her boyfriend knew how much he loved her, she was learning how much she deserved to love herself—regardless of her appearance or her accomplishments. That's a win in my book.

But there was something else that I hoped Casey would get out of our work together. I wanted to reconnect her with her joy—something I feared she had lost somewhere long ago in her childhood. As anxiety often drives us to do, we grow up too quickly and leave behind the folly and the fun because it feels frivolous. It lacks purpose. And that's exactly why we need it even more.

Maybe you too have staved off your joy. We don't allow for the vulnerability of laughter or heartfelt tears because we believe it leaves us defenseless. We see expression of emotion as weakness instead of a moment of connection. We've internalized that adults don't goof off, cry, or laugh (unless we're inebriated and therefore less likely to worry about inhibitions).

I know that most of us want to reconnect to our joy, though. Part of why nostalgia is so powerful is because it feels like one of the few vessels through which we can tap back into that childlike wonder we miss. It's why we love watching babies, because they unabashedly have permission to do all the things we wish we could do—laugh, cry, play—without judgment.

What if you allowed yourself to loosen the grip, though? What if you didn't judge yourself for laughing so hard that people turned around because they heard you? What if you danced at a wedding and others noticed you? What if? What if? What if? And to that I say, "So what. So what. So what." Your anxiety doesn't need to have a death grip on your joy. Let yourself love what you love without putting parameters on it.

LET'S TAKE AN OPPORTUNITY TO DEFINE SOME OF THE WAYS THAT YOU COULD INCORPORATE MORE PLAY INTO YOUR LIFE. TELL ME, WHAT SPARKS YOUR CHILDLIKE JOY?

1. _____

2. _____

3. _____

4. _____

5. _____

Come back to play. Find those things that you loved to do as a child and rediscover them. Find new things that spark your interest and get lost in them. Not everything needs to be done for productivity's sake. Not everything needs to have a purpose. Get lost in time and just enjoy something for the pure sake of enjoyment. When you can be free to live out your joy, your anxiety won't have such a stronghold on your life. Yes, you may still feel anxious sometimes when you're trying something new. The key is that you're not letting your anxiety stop you altogether. You're coming back to that little kid inside who just wants to play.

CHAPTER EIGHT

SUPPORTING YOUR FELLOW SURFERS FROM AFAR

Sometimes you can tell a client hasn't slept well in a few days. With Jessie, it looked as if she hadn't slept in a few weeks. A queer, agnostic, transgender, Latinx woman, she told me that she had barely gotten a few hours of rest because her best friend from college, whom we'll call Tony, was imprisoned a few months ago because of a reported burglary. According to Jessie, what began as an alcohol addiction for Tony evolved into a cocaine problem. He had begun acting erratically over the past six months and Jessie told me she had been worried sick about him. While she felt that she should help her friend, she said the situation really devolved when she learned that he was arrested for breaking and entering, with a gun. Now that he was in jail and couldn't afford bail, Tony was all she could think about. Not only was she trying to gather funds for his bail, she also began skipping her classes, ignoring her other friends, and hardly sleeping because she never knew when Tony might call from jail. She told me that she felt like death, but she didn't want to "let Tony down." She came to me in hopes that I could help her help her friend. I had another purpose, though: to help her help *herself.*

I realize that many of you, like Jessie, are mini therapists in the making. You could have completed an internship by now with all the hours you've done giving therapy sessions at three in the morning. And while it's beyond generous of you to support your friends and family in this way, it's not sustainable. That's why I had to include this chapter. I'm writing this not only so that you can help those around you who are struggling—but also so you can protect your own well-being. When you're working overtime for the people in your life, it's a fast-track road to burnout. And while you started out as the lifeguard, you can quickly find yourself drowning if you're not careful.

You're probably thinking of someone you're worried about right now as you read this chapter. There is likely no greater pain than watching our friends and family suffer. Sometimes it's worse than bearing our own burdens. And whether another's behavior is intentional or unintentional, it rips us to our core. To feel some semblance of control, we often want to jump in and take action because we feel utterly powerless watching destruction right before our eyes.

Here's the thing, though. We can't control the choices that other people make in their lives. Jessie couldn't control that Tony robbed someone's home or that he started using cocaine. While some people judged Jessie for keeping her friendship with Tony after this happened, she held on to something that many people around her struggled to see: the both/and. She was able to see his beautiful heart and not just the tough choices he had made. She knew that Tony was still a good person who had made some questionable decisions—but that didn't make him a bad person altogether. I found this compassion from Jessie to be a beautiful thing, especially when so many others around Tony had cut him off—and her as well, because she continued to be his friend.

However, I became concerned for Jessie when I saw how she was starting to abandon her well-being to be there for him. She told me that she thought she was a "bad friend" if she didn't sacrifice as much as possible for Tony. I had to remind her of her own both/and: she could still be a good friend and practice self-care. Because as hard as it was for Jessie to sit with, she was realizing that we can't control what our parents, our friends, or our family members do. All that she could control was herself and how she looked after her own welfare.

Perhaps you can relate. You too may have a parent who struggles with alcoholism. A friend who regularly threatens suicide. A sibling who has an eating disorder and refuses to get help. All of these are self-harming behaviors in their own right. It's like watching a plane crash in slow motion. You can't stop it. It's hard to watch.

When I'm reminded of this, I can't help but think back to my Uncle Matt, my Grandma Joan's youngest child, and his battle with alcoholism. While he was once the life of the party when we were young, we watched him devolve into a jaundiced man who couldn't put the bottle down. Our family chased him. I remember my cousins and me sitting in the back seat of a car at a nearby motel where our dads (his brothers) tried to convince him to go to rehab. He said adamantly, "No." Demanded, "Leave me alone." Even though we kept knocking, Uncle Matt ended up dying by himself in a hotel room at forty-three years old. I remember we got the call at my voice recital when I was thirteen. I wish I could tell you that we were surprised but we weren't. It still broke our hearts. I'll never forget hugging my Grandma Joan in the church parking lot and crying together. Her son was gone. All these years later, I still think of him every time I drive by that motel.

My loss of Uncle Matt left a mark. I don't drink much myself because it reminds me of what our family went through. I also don't work with clients who use substances extensively because it just hurts too much. Even though I'm well aware that relapse is part of the picture when clients are in recovery, I take it too hard when someone uses again after years of sobriety.

If you're resonating with any of this, I know you've been carrying a lot. Maybe you blame yourself for not answering the phone that one time. Or you think it's your fault that your family member relapsed because you got into a fight. My hope is that in reading this, you can unburden yourself of the guilt that you may be carrying.

I want to say this loud and clear: you are not responsible for the choices that another person makes.

You cannot always control whether someone decides to harm themselves. You cannot be inside their brain. You can't control their body and what they do to it. Unless someone is hospitalized because they are a risk to themselves or others, or they are a minor, there is only so much you can do. I know it can feel like you could always do a "little more," but, honestly, the little more that you can do is look after yourself. At the end of the day, it's up to the person in distress to get the help and implement it. They have to be the one to take the step, especially if it's going to last. They have to want it for themselves.

A NEW WAVE TO RIDE:

Do you find yourself frequently worrying about someone and wishing there was more you could do to control the situation? How can you hold loving someone *and* loving yourself at the same time so that you don't forgo your own well-being in the process?

WHEN YOUR BOARD IS SINKING

Like Jessie, you may find that you've added everyone and their mothers' problems to your plate. Jessie was so preoccupied hoping to take care of Tony that she had completely forgotten to take care of herself. When I asked her about this, she told me that it would have been inconsiderate to look after herself when Tony had "much bigger problems" to face.

I reminded her that she had the capacity to give herself permission to both care about Tony and look after herself. In fact, caring for herself was a way to show Tony that she wasn't giving up on either of them. It could even inspire him to do the same for himself.

She told me that she hadn't thought of it that way.

Like Jessie, a lot of us stop living our own lives because we feel like we need to constantly look after someone else's. To be fair, this is where the system has failed us. We have not provided nearly enough resources so that people have equitable access to care. People can't find therapists or can't afford them (pro tip: go to a university training clinic for sliding scale options). For those struggling with SMI (serious mental illness), our system often leaves folks with two options: prison or hospitalization. Many family members and friends are *forced* into providing long-term care because there is nowhere else for struggling folks to go to.

I used to see this all the time when I worked at UCLA in the Center for the Assessment and Prevention of Prodromal States (CAPPS), where we were studying signs of early-onset psychosis and its progression. Looking into exasperated parents' eyes, we'd cover the list of resources and admittedly, they were limited. Sometimes they would say, "I've tried all of this already. Is this all?" And my answer would unfortunately be "Yes. I wish there were more." I'd then proceed to call for a hospital bed for the client who was in psychosis, only to be told that there were none and the family would have to drive two hours to find a bed for the night before the client could get transferred. If that sounds exhausting, that's because it is.

A couple of years of this and it's understandable why many people experience houselessness or end up in jail, like Tony. Without the privilege of families who can take care of them, it's not uncommon that at eighteen years old or a few years down the line, clients end up left to their own devices. Especially if they don't have access to therapy or don't stick to a medication regimen, then drugs, alcohol, and other unsafe coping tools can get picked up as a means of survival. Whether in a state of psychosis, on a bender, these folks can engage in behaviors that affirm the worst-held stereotypes about mental illness, including that people are dangerous and not to be trusted.[99,100,101]

When our worst fears come true and we see headlines in the news, we can easily point our fingers and say that the parents were not "doing enough." Yet I invite anyone to live a week in the life of a caretaker, especially a family member or friend who is trying to help someone who is noncompliant with treatment. It's not always a cakewalk. Sometimes, it's unsustainable. When caretakers make the tough decision that they need to set boundaries in their lives, we can see the aftermath of folks ending up on the street or in jail. We shake our heads, wondering what the heck happened.

Well, here's what happened. Instead of supporting these clients and their families who may have struggled for years, our health care system just waited for trouble to ensue. As the National Alliance on Mental Illness says, "You should fear the broken system, not the people it has failed."[102] Whether it's someone driving under the influence and hitting someone fatally, or an at-risk youth who got involved with drugs (like Tony), we point our fingers at the parents or the person's peers instead of considering how we are systemically dropping the ball. It's not only that we're not doing enough—we're making it way too easy for these problems to perpetuate. Realistically, though, we also cannot monitor every move of someone we're concerned about. If we're already at that point, then we know a larger framework of support should have been brought in beforehand.

Sadly, that support just isn't always there. We don't always have safe and effective places for these people to go. We could write a whole separate book on the debate on deinstitutionalization, but the truth of the matter is, we need more support for individuals and the caregivers who surround them. Instead of blaming others, like Jessie, for not "fixing" the problem or "noticing the signs," we need to provide more education on bystander interventions while destigmatizing accessing services. We need to have larger conversations about how to finance housing and staff for those who need daily support. Don't get me wrong, I'm all for a recovery-based model of care where we empower the person to take as much ownership over their life as possible.[103] But until then, it's no wonder caretakers experience tremendous anxiety— they inherently know that the onus of responsibility may very well fall on them rather than the person who actually invoked harm. Furthermore, if they don't care—then who does? This was the question that kept Jessie up at night when she would wait for Tony's call, which never seemed to come.

I know that for many of you, worrying about someone else is practically your full-time job. You stress about whether your loved one will go to their therapy appointment today or ditch. Did they take their pills and refill their prescription? Do they have access to sharp objects? Did they relapse? It's exhausting to drown in those thoughts—especially when there is only so much that you can do.

This is where we come back to it: empowered acceptance.

I want to switch it up this time, though, and instead of starting with acceptance, as we often do, let's begin with the empowerment piece. I don't want you to read this chapter and walk away believing that you need to give up on your loved ones. Quite the opposite. I want you to be wholly empowered in doing what you can at the pace that you can. If you have the bandwidth to support someone in a way that motivates them to take care of themselves, by all means, go for it.

Let's break down the difference, though, between empowered support and enabled support.

ENABLED SUPPORT	EMPOWERED SUPPORT
Listening to your friend's challenges for weeks (and months) on end but being too afraid to recommend they see a therapist. You don't want to offend them, after all.	Listening to your friend's challenges and offering to help them find a therapist to support them long-term. If they can't afford therapy, you can help them find a mentor or spiritual leader who can offer some free guidance. In the meantime, establish set times to speak with your friend about what's going on so that you are setting boundaries around your time and not feeling burnt-out.

ENABLED SUPPORT	EMPOWERED SUPPORT
Noticing that your sister rarely eats and watching this pattern play out for years. Because you want to keep the peace in the relationship, you don't say anything.	Telling your sister that you're concerned about her eating behaviors and sharing that you think it would be helpful for her to get an evaluation. Offer to go along with her to get her bloodwork done and/or go to the hospital together.
Checking in daily to see whether your spouse took their medication. "Did you take it?" One hour later: "Did you take it?"	Helping your spouse with regularly taking their medication by having it out in an easy-to-see place.
Asking your partner for the play-by-play of what they discussed in therapy and asking whether you came up in session.	Driving your partner to a therapy session and asking how they're doing without prying for more information.
Buying alcohol and other substances and staying out late with your friend to help them numb their pain.	Cooking healthy meals with your friend, inviting them for a walk, and developing new self-care practices as a team.
Allowing your friend to stay with you for months on end, even though you resent it and it's causing problems in your other relationships.	Letting a friend stay with you for a few weeks while they get back on their feet and then having a plan for them to get their own place.

When we're offering enabled support, it's typically because we want to control the person or situation through love. We feel that if we check in enough, we just might prevent any pain from happening. While we don't want our loved ones to be in pain, we have to ask ourselves: Is it actually more about avoiding our *own* pain? Whether it's the pain of guilt, anger, unpredictability—our controlling behavior is often a balm to protect ourselves, not just the person who is struggling.

It can also be a lot easier to look at someone else's hardships rather than our own. It's not uncommon for families to have an "identified patient," where everyone else can put their time and attention toward the "sick one" so that they rarely have to face their own demons.[104] This is something we all can get curious about. Are we running toward others so that we don't have to run with ourselves? I certainly saw this hold true with Jessie. As a woman who had fought diligently to get herself into a great undergraduate program, she was quick to let Tony's setback veer her off her own course. She was so preoccupied with his problems that she felt it excused her own neglect. She thought this was just what good friends did.

Thankfully we were able to reroute. Leaning into her own empowerment, Jessie became more aware of what she could and couldn't do for Tony. She could assist him with legal resources, and she did so. She could be there for him as a friend to answer the phone when the timing worked out. But wait for hours on end for a phone to ring that rarely did? Or miss out on sleep on the off chance he would call her? Or add to the large amount in student loans that she already had to help pay off his bail? No longer. After talking in therapy about the dialectic, and holding that she could both be a caring friend and protect her own well-being, Jessie explained to Tony what she could and couldn't do. This wasn't personal. She let him know that her own health was suffering, and she had to make time for herself if she was going to continue with her program. Thankfully, Tony understood. In fact, he was exceedingly supportive of Jessie and told her that he wanted nothing but the best for her. But if he'd guilted her for not bailing him out or being there every waking (and unwaking) minute? As I shared with Jessie—this would've been helpful data to make note of. This is not what a fair friendship would look like.

If you have your own friend or loved one who guilts or shames you for protecting your own well-being, you may very well have a shark swimming in your waters. You shouldn't be punished for making time for your self-care. If you've been there for them through the ups and downs and then they blame you the second you put a boundary up, no can do. That's often the makings of an unsustainable relationship. You're not a personal assistant for someone, waiting at their beck and call the second they need you. Not even therapists operate like that. People need to respect your limits and it starts by you respecting your own.

WHEN IT'S TIME FOR SOMEONE TO SWIM ON THEIR OWN

Once you've leaned into empowerment and you've done what you can, then the acceptance piece emerges. I'd argue this is the hardest part. It's challenging enough to accept our own struggles; it's even harder to accept when someone continues to choose a difficult path. While I'm not a mother yet, I imagine it's akin to what I hear many mothers say: the pain of letting your child go off into the world, knowing that they will get hurt, and knowing that you cannot protect them—it is a pain unlike any other. And yet, it's something we must accept.

We've all seen what happens when mothers emotionally suffocate their children. Those children can become needy, complacent, rebellious, angry, or anxious, among a whole host of other presentations, because they haven't been given ample room to skin their knees and make messes of themselves. Sometimes we have to fall flat on our faces to feel the sting on our skin. Being told to watch out is not enough. We have to know it and feel it for ourselves.

So many of us are trying to block pain for our friends and family members in a whole host of ways. We see all the potential places where it could go wrong, and we feel that it's our job to step in. We equate protection and prevention with caring. While we don't want to let our friend knowingly walk into a major mistake (like marry an abusive person or get sucked into a cult—which seriously happens), we also have to let our loved ones make their own decisions and face the consequences of their choices. They need to take their own steps—it's not our job to interfere. And if we're being honest with ourselves, we likely want this same respect in return. After all, if you've ever had someone give unsolicited advice or you've heard from someone who "knows best," it's usually not the most appreciated feedback. You want to be trusted to captain your own ship.

What's worse, by trying to help others avert their own pain, we magnify our own. This kind of pain is even worse because it's not even done by our own hands—it's completely contingent on what our loved ones decide to do. We then box ourselves in, trying our hardest to be exactly what the other person needs us to be. What someone chooses to do should not be contingent on your behavior. And if it is—you do not need to buy into the myth that it's your fault that you "weren't there" for them. This is manipulative behavior in its purest form.

What your loved ones choose to do is not a reflection on you. No matter what happens: it's not your fault.

This is something I reminded Jessie of regularly. She was so afraid that Tony would continue to suffer if she wasn't there to constantly try to save him. The truth of the matter, though, was that neither she nor I could prevent his pain. Tony had to endure the consequences of his actions. Only he could be the one to decide to change. His hand couldn't be forced. No amount of friendship or money from Jessie could guarantee that he would make different choices moving forward. She could of course let him know that she was there for him, but she ultimately had to accept that Tony had to live his own life—she couldn't live it for him.

Part of acceptance is acknowledging that others may continue to inflict pain on themselves, even if they know it pains you to see it. Most of the time, they're not doing this with malicious intent. Their goal isn't to hurt you. It's just that sometimes, their pain is so great that it ricochets onto others—and you might be in the line of fire. While we can't always stop the fire from coming, we can at least get some protective gear. More on that later.

For the person using or harming themselves, they often feel a sense of powerlessness similar to yours. They may very well want the maladaptive behaviors to change and yet, even with the best of intentions, the cycle continues. In fact, 75 percent of those struggling with addiction will relapse within the first year.[105] One study found that 35 to 41 percent of eating disorder recovery clients relapse after completing treatment.[106] Even if the desire to get better is there, sometimes willpower is not enough. There can be a constant battle with biology, and when this happens, it doesn't mean that your friend or family member doesn't love you enough to want to recover. All the love in the world can be there—it's just that the addiction and/or the mental illness is that powerful. It's likely not about you—even though it can feel so personal.

At the same time, it's not foolish to hope that it can get better. While I said about 75 percent of people relapse in the first year, the CDC and the National Institute on Drug Abuse in 2020 found that 75 percent also go on to fully recover.[107] That's promising news given that 9 percent of adults in the United States are currently in recovery from a substance-use disorder.[108] There are also hopeful statistics when it comes to suicidality. Nine out of ten people who attempt suicide will survive and not die by suicide at a later time.[109] This shows that suicidal ideation does not last forever and the intensity of the pain can pass.

It's impossible to predict the future, though. While we don't even know what our own future holds, we surely don't know what lies ahead for our loved ones. This unpredictability of possible pain can derail us and yet, we have to sit with the reality of it. That's what acceptance is. On the note of suicide, take the fact that 60 percent of people who die by suicide did not make a previous attempt.[110] Additionally, many suicide attempts are unplanned, with 48 to 85 percent of attempters disclosing that they experienced a sudden inclination to harm themselves and did not plan their attempt in advance.[111,112] This speaks to the impulsivity that often comes with self-harm. While there can certainly be warning signs, it can be so easy for people to either hide those signs or not notice them themselves. In fact, more than half of people who die by suicide were never diagnosed with a mental illness or saw a mental health provider.[113] So while you may be sitting there, blaming yourself for "not seeing it sooner," it's likely that the person didn't even see it for themselves. With people lacking the tools to cope, the tide can turn very quickly. The pain—and their desire to make that pain go away—can be all they see. When someone isn't willing to accept their pain—whether it's from shame, embarrassment, or sadness—it can get passed on to us instead. This unwanted transfer is typically unintentional, but we fear it nonetheless.

We also can take someone's behavior so personally when really, it's someone's biology getting the better of them. Because we have been numbed to our pain for so long, many of us don't realize when we're struggling until it smacks us in the face. If we get hit with a sudden stressor, like a breakup, a firing, or a large financial loss, that pain can be like a tidal wave that topples us completely over. We forget that there are smaller and less intense waves behind it. In these moments of severe distress, our brains may be working against us. Given that the brain's frontal lobe doesn't finish developing until we're twenty-five, all of our faculties that help us with self-control, considering consequences, and holding empathy for others may not be in check.[114] Even if you're over twenty-five, when that amygdala gets set off, whether it's from anger, sadness, or fear, you can quickly lose hope that it can get better. That's why when someone is feeling suicidal, wanting to use again, or considering any kind of self-harm, they're not trying to push their pain onto you. They're just trying to make the pain disappear.

That's why you need to remember: what someone chooses to do with their life is not your fault. You do not control their brain (in fact, it'd be scary if you did). You may be kicking yourself, telling yourself you should have seen the signs or done something more. This isn't in your hands, though—and it never was. It's not your job to prevent someone else's suicide, recidivism, or relapse. You can help if you can—but the onus of responsibility does not fall on you. It falls on the person living and breathing in their own body. That is their freedom of choice, just as you have yours. This is where empowerment comes back in.

WHEN THE RIDE NEEDS TO CHANGE AND YOU'VE GOT TO SAY SO

Empowerment can present itself in many different ways when it comes to our relationships. It can look like empowering others to take care of themselves. It can mean that we're empowered in loving and protecting ourselves, especially when someone keeps inflicting pain on us. It can also look like being empowered to lean into the tough conversations that we'd rather avoid when we're concerned about someone.

Many of us unknowingly enable our friends and loved ones because we don't want to share the tough feedback that they've hurt us or that we're worried about them. We're so scared to rock the boat and exacerbate their distress that we swallow our own frustration. And yet, in doing so, we are perpetuating our pain and their pain further. If you're feeling worried, angry, or disappointed, your feelings are valid. You deserve to have your own opportunity to express your experience. It doesn't mean that by sharing, you will change what the person chooses to do with their life, but at least you're seeing the relationship through a much more honest lens. It's hard for resentment to build up if you're giving yourself a release valve.

I have a feeling you've been thinking about someone throughout this entire chapter, so I want to offer some tools that may be helpful if you're considering having a conversation with them. It starts by getting a general sense of how a person feels about their behavior. Known as the Stages of Change Model, originally developed by James Prochaska and Carlo DiClemente, this framework is a helpful way to conceptualize how motivated someone may be to change.[115,116] I'll briefly break down each stage and as I do so, notice where various friends and family members (as well as you yourself) lie in this lineup.

1. **Precontemplation:** This is when someone is in denial about their problem. They're not motivated to make a change because they don't see the need for making one. They can be defensive about their behavior and they see more pros than cons with their current setup.

2. **Contemplation:** The person is aware that a problem exists but they're unsure whether they'd like to make a change. They may feel ambivalent and indecisive about how to proceed. They can see the value of choosing differently but it's unclear whether the discomfort of change is worth it to them.

3. **Preparation:** They acknowledge that a problem exists and they're looking to gather resources to help sustain a change. They realize it will be uncomfortable to choose a new response but the pros now outweigh the cons. They may even feel excited and hopeful about a new response pattern.

4. **Action:** This is when the change actually happens. The person receives support and shares how they are making different behavioral choices. It's not just talking the talk—it's walking the walk. A mix of emotions can occur during this time. It can be harder than they thought but they may also feel proud of themselves. It may be a constant battle within themselves but they're in the fight.

5. **Relapse:** A natural part of the process, we should expect that the path to change will never be linear. The pros of the past behavior lured them back while they may be forgetting all the cons that came along with it. There is a lot of learning that happens during a relapse, and it doesn't mean that progress is completely derailed.

6. **Maintenance:** After making the initial change, the person sustains their progress and integrates this new behavior. They have found alternative coping skills and they are motivated to continue on their new path. The pros of change now outweigh the pros of their past behavior.

What's helpful about knowing (generally) where someone sits in the Stages of Change Model is that it can inform how you have a conversation with the person. If we assume how ready someone is, many of us can misstep by jumping in with an action-oriented conversation when the person is actually in the precontemplation stage. Or we can jump to the worst-case scenario when someone relapses and assume they're back to the precontemplation stage. In reality, it may just be a slipup and they have every intention of sustaining the change.

That's why motivational interviewing questions can be one of the most invaluable tools you use when you're supporting friends and family. The idea is that you can ask nonaccusatory questions that help the person come to their own conclusions, rather than being forced into a choice that they're not ready to make. After all, it's one thing to make someone feel guilty for their behavior and then they change out of resentment. It's another to help someone build their own innate desire for a different path.

Here are some examples of questions that you can use when you'd like to support someone in making a change. Every time "behavior" is listed, replace it with the specific concern (substance use, depression, self-harm, etc.) that you are worried about.

1. How would you say your current behavior is impacting you?
2. How do you feel about the behavior?
3. How would you feel if your current behavior didn't change?
4. On a scale from 1 to 10, how ready do you feel to make a change regarding your current behavior?
5. How do you think making this change would improve your life, if at all?
6. What do you see getting in the way of making this change?
7. If you'd like my support, how can I help you make this change?
8. If you decided to change, what would your next steps look like?
9. What hasn't worked about making a change in the past?
10. How should we plan to communicate about this current behavior moving forward?

As you go through these questions, you'll want to integrate the OARS tool. This stands for a set of skills that includes asking

open-ended questions, **affirming** the person's experience, offering **reflective** listening, and **summarizing** what has been shared.[117] This helps the person express where they currently stand as you engage in a nonjudgmental way.

You'll notice that all of these questions lean more into curiosity than accusation. When you come in with an open stance, the person has room to reflect. If you go in hot and make it about you, the conversation is likely not going to go how you want. No one likes to feel attacked. When the finger-wagging comes at us, it's a common defense to lie, get angry, or dig our heels in even more. Even if someone says they'll change, it's unclear whether they want to improve to get you off their back or because they genuinely want to improve for themselves. If you can sit with your discomfort and not let your pain push the conversation forward, there's room for the person's real answers to bubble up. It's a lot easier for someone to buy into change when they've come to the conclusion themselves.

For the caretakers, you have to start by understanding where you are at in your own process as well. When Jessie took the time to sit with her own feelings, rather than just focus solely on Tony, she realized just how angry and sad she was.

She lamented, "I hate that he did this to me. Even more, I hate that he did this to himself. I just want to rage at him."

"I can understand that. You were having such a great time together and then he made a different choice that derailed your plans. You were just so excited to enjoy college together."

I followed up, "But do you think raging at him would actually get you anywhere?"

"A part of me wishes it would but if I'm being honest, I don't think it would. I'm sure he's struggling enough as it is. Getting shame from me wouldn't change anything."

This is where Jessie and I practiced some role-plays to help her assess where Tony was at in the Stages of Change. She could integrate some of the motivational interview questions to see how much he wanted to shift his behaviors. Rather than judge his behavior, she tried to keep an open mind and let him explain for himself why he did the things that he did, as well as how he felt about what he did.

When she eventually had a conversation with him using the techniques, she told me that it was enlightening. While she had assumed he was in the precontemplation stage, she saw how the arrest had shifted things for him. Tony shared his "wake-up call" that happened in jail. He had hopes for a great career, just like Jessie, but his drug use had derailed him faster than he thought possible. Getting arrested made him see how quickly things could turn. He saw Jessie's life and wanted what she had. While she was getting her life back on track by going to classes again and developing some new friendships, he was feeling left behind. He decided that no high from any drug was worth the risk of losing it all. He said aloud to her that he was ready to get sober.

Jessie cried as she told me about this news.

"I had given up hope that things could change. I worried that he would be a lost cause. But I'm so glad that I came to the conversation with an open mind. I could tell that he was telling himself what he wanted to do. It was his agenda—not my own."

It worked out for Jessie this time around. It might not have in another set of circumstances. That is how empowered acceptance works. You show up empowered to lean into the conversation—and you accept that you may not be happy with the outcome. You accept that you do not have control over what someone chooses to do and you are empowered to still live your life in spite of what's out of your hands. By letting go and still leaning in, that's what Jessie was doing in her friendship with Tony. Her well-being was no longer contingent on his sobriety.

Whether you stage an intervention with a loved one or friend is up to you. There's mixed research on the effectiveness of interventions. Some say that strong conversations with boundary setting, including ultimatums (e.g., "You cannot live here if you are going to continue to use"), are necessary, while others recommend a gentler entry point so that the person may be less defensive. I won't encourage being in one camp or the other—I think it's highly dependent on your relationship with the person, how long this has been going on, and how your own mental health is faring. If you have the bandwidth and you're just starting out with someone, a less confrontational conversation may be the best approach. But if you're at your wit's end and you're feeling disrespected, manipulated, and/or unsafe, by all means protect your welfare first and foremost. You are not an unloving parent, friend, or family member because you discontinue letting a person take advantage of a situation. For example, if Tony had been guilting Jessie into giving him money or pressuring her to use with him, we'd have had a different conversation entirely about learning how to set and maintain appropriate boundaries so that she could keep herself physically, mentally, and emotionally safe. The key point no matter what: you need to model what it looks like to have self-respect.

I realize how entirely anxiety-provoking this all is. It can feel like you lose either way. Even if they say they want to change, you may worry that it won't last. When they don't care to make a different choice, you worry that you'll never be able to convince them otherwise. No matter how hard you pull the rope in this tug-of-war, it's not your battle to win. You can't save anyone. We have to learn how to let go. No amount of worrying is going to resolve the situation. Resources can help. Conversations can motivate. But ultimately, each person decides for themselves if they want to make and sustain a change.

PROTECTING YOUR OWN SURFBOARD

When you're watching someone actively hurt themselves or derail their lives, it is really hard to sit with. This is where you've got to love yourself a little (or a lot) harder. When you're so worried about someone else, there's little time to consider how you're doing. Being a caretaker (or a constant fretter) is a full-time job if you allow it to be. I've seen so many people develop anxiety disorders and come down with depressive episodes because they're so immersed in someone else's pain. You need to look after yourself. It's painful enough to see one person suffer—you don't need to get so far pulled down that your life completely unravels as well.

Some of us think we don't truly love someone if we don't get sucked into their chaos. That's called enmeshment, friend. Codependency, even. When you do not allow yourself to thrive because someone else isn't, it doesn't make the situation better. It stagnates it. Like with Jessie, when she was forgoing her own well-being, it didn't make Tony's situation any better. It was only making her situation worse. It's a trope that you may have heard by now but it's worth reiterating: you have to put your own oxygen mask on first before you can help someone else.

I hope this is a wake-up call to take care of yourself. There are so many ways that you can get support. Here are just a few ideas:

- Join a NAMI (National Alliance on Mental Illness) group if you have a family member struggling with a mental illness and/ or addiction, as well as other support groups such as Al-Anon (they specifically help those with family members experiencing alcohol abuse).
- Go to therapy for yourself to process your experience.
- Hold boundaries around sleep, exercise, nutrition, and hydration.
- Understand your budget and hold firm to what money you need for your own livelihood.
- Talk to someone removed from the situation to get your own support and an outside perspective.
- Get community support through a worship service, sound bath retreat, or a meditation group.
- Get a massage or do a yoga class.
- Participate in a group walk or fundraiser to process, heal, and connect with other folks who can resonate with your experience (for example, the Out of the Darkness Walk is specifically for those impacted by suicide).

More than anything, you need to allow yourself the space to emotionally process what you've gone through (or are continuing to go through). Feel the sadness, the disappointment, and the fear. Feel the *anger*. Sometimes we can feel like we have to suppress this particular emotion, especially when we're afraid it will make the other person lash out or run away. Problematic behaviors perpetuate, though, when everyone is willing to placate the person who is inflicting harm on themselves or others. You deserve to have your own emotional experience, and whether or not you share it with the person who made you feel that way, you do need some opportunity to express what's coming up for you. Don't keep the toxicity of your heartache inside. We'll talk in chapter 10 about what happens when you do.

I know we wish the future could be clearer. We can make ourselves sick as we mull over the unknown. I don't have the answers for you, and neither do you. Neither does the person you're worried about. They don't know what they are going to decide to do next week, just as we don't know our own path ahead, either. We can have intention. That's certainly worth something. But sometimes circumstances are outside our control. Sometimes the cards are drawn in such a way that people make choices that shatter us—and shatter them as well. It's not what anyone wants, but that is life. The pain is not inevitable . . . but it's possible.

Life is a series of both/ands. It's the ambivalence of wanting to get better and still succumbing to the momentary sips of sweetness that turn sour. We can wait in anticipation for that fallout moment to come . . . or we can trust.

It's not about trusting other people. That can be a fool's game. Everyone messes up and if you're hoping your loved ones will have a perfect track record, you're going to end up inescapably disappointed.

I'm talking about trusting yourself. Trust that you can handle the pain if and when it comes. You don't need to make yourself sick with worry waiting for a shoe to drop. It might and it might not. You don't need to guilt yourself that you "could have done more." Sure, you could do more and even still, that may never be enough. Trust that when someone makes a choice that hurts you, it's rarely about you. You may tell yourself, "If they really loved me, they would stop." It's not that they don't love you—it's that they're not ready to be grossly uncomfortable by making a change in their lives. They can't handle the pain of shifting their behavior, at least not right now, and so they choose the pain of continuing their destructive habits instead. I know it's so hard to watch—I've had to watch myself from the back seat of that car in the motel parking lot when I was a kid.

I'm glad to say that Jessie realized that she could care vehemently for Tony and not be responsible for making his life look different. He was responsible for changing his outcome, not she. I know you may be reading this and wondering what happened to Tony. Did he get sober? Did he get out of jail?

I don't actually know. Jessie decided while we were working together that she wanted to study abroad in Ireland. Even though she initially felt some guilt about going abroad while Tony was still waiting for his trial, we worked through how she deserved to take on this opportunity that she was excited about. As she got ready to fly across the Atlantic, we decided to conclude treatment. After all, she had accomplished the goal that she didn't know she needed to set: she was taking care of herself. There were no more excuses and there was no more time to waste. She was learning how to control what she could: her future and hers alone. Everything else, including Tony's path, she accepted was beyond her control. She still cared, but she now cared just as much about what was best for her. I haven't heard from her since.

The truth is that the only behavior you can change is your own. Choose to take better care of yourself. Mend your heart if it's broken. Give yourself a chance to steady your nerves if you're stretched thin. If you've been caught in someone else's rip current for a long time, you're not soulless to swim away. It's self-preservation. You owe it to yourself—and everyone else around you who wants to see you thrive—to get in calmer waters. You can still love someone and watch them from afar. Give yourself that permission so that you can just keep swimming.

CHAPTER NINE

THE SELF-CARE STRATEGIES THAT HELP YOU STAY AFLOAT

When I met with Suma, a South Asian, Hindu, straight, cisgender woman, I felt a strong connection to her. Similar to my own experience with anxiety, her stress manifested physically. When she talked about feeling trapped in her body and being afraid of when the next unexpected panic attack would strike, I knew how she felt. Part of what upset Suma so much was that there wasn't a direct trigger for her symptoms. There was no identifiable trauma, no phobias, no social anxiety—just pure anxiety that made her feel like her body was under attack. When there's no clear cue, as in Suma's case, this can be even more frustrating, as the unpredictability of symptoms can feel even more distressing.

When this is the case, we often come back to the body and how we can restore it. For this reason, this chapter focuses on all the ways that we can improve our anxiety by lovingly caring for our bodies as a self-care practice. As much as the cognitive work makes a difference (which we've covered all throughout the book so far), we often have to reconnect to our bodies and minds through physical and emotional healing that goes beyond the textbook. Because so many of us are afraid of our bodies' reactions to anxiety, rebuilding a relationship with our physicality—where we see our bodies as healers rather than tormentors—is essential.

A key reminder: care for clients, including for you, is not a one-size-fits-all approach. Even though Westernized medicine can make it seem like therapy and psychiatry (aka medication) are the two best treatment routes, there are so many other modalities that hold possibilities for healing. While I'm all for evidence-based practices, such as cognitive behavioral therapy (CBT) and the integration of pharmaceuticals, if it's clinically indicated, I ultimately like to support what's going to be most helpful for my client (as long as the client is not at immediate risk for harming themselves or someone else—this is when the most empirically supported interventions are warranted). In most cases, treatment includes the client making an informed decision about what will serve them best. That's why I'd be remiss if I didn't include this chapter for you. It's crucial to consider everything available in your tool kit.

Where to begin? We need to start by understanding what our bodies are trying to tell us. That's why I'm such an advocate for getting our bloodwork done. It's not uncommon for me to see clients spend thousands of dollars on therapy when the root of their anxiety is tied to a hormonal imbalance or a nutritional deficiency. If a client is presenting with any symptoms that could be biologically driven (insomnia, low energy, or gastrointestinal issues, for example), I almost always recommend they get a blood panel done with either their general physician or a naturopathic doctor so that we can understand at baseline how their body is doing.

There can be invaluable answers in your bloodwork that could be the ticket to your recovery. So many of us keep ourselves in a state of purgatory because we're afraid of the pain of a needle or we're worried we won't be able to handle the news if something is actually wrong. But it's when you've empowered yourself with this data that you can take meaningful action. You do not need to keep yourself in the cycle of worry, wondering why, for example, you're constantly feeling foggy or exhausted, why your skin is frequently breaking out, or why you struggle to get an erection (yep, we're going there, because too many men suffer in silence about this one). There may be some easily explainable answers, and it all starts with getting your bloodwork done.

I've seen the power of this in my own life. While I've grappled with emetophobia for basically as long as I can remember, I was finding that my panic attacks were spiraling out of control in recent years. If I felt like I was trapped (in a plane, on a bus, or even stuck inside a booth at a restaurant), it wasn't uncommon for me to eventually start shaking, feel incredibly nauseous, and have difficulty breathing. My brain would start thinking of all the worst-case scenarios, especially, "What will happen if I throw up right here at the table?" It was getting harder and harder to deny my symptoms and I wondered whether others were catching on. I was at a breaking point in the fall of 2020. While I'd done exposure therapy for these panic attacks (as I covered in chapter 4), it wasn't until I began seeing a naturopathic doctor who recommended that I get my bloodwork done that things started to turn around.

Soon after, I learned that I had vitamin D, vitamin B_{12}, and magnesium deficiencies. Interestingly, as I began doing the research, I learned the impact that such imbalances can have on the body, particularly when it comes to creating an internal cocktail that will get you emotionally intoxicated on a daily basis with anxious distress. For someone like me who had been drinking that blend for years and was starting to believe that's just how it would always be, this information about the power of vitamin and mineral balances was beyond enlightening. Given that I had started to become resigned to my anxiety and panic, it was the first time in a long time that I felt a sense of hope.

Now, that's not to say that the cognitive work isn't also essential. I've done a lot to manage how I respond to my anxious thoughts, and exposure and response prevention therapy was still quite helpful (and it's the first-line intervention for those with panic). But given how life-changing it has been to get my overall body back in balance through supplements and nutrition, I have to share this part of the equation with you. Getting my body in a more homeostatic state has made my anxiety threshold much higher. This means that it takes a lot more to trigger a panic attack, whereas before, when I was experiencing nutritional deficiencies, it took so little to set off the symptoms. Now I find that I have far fewer anxious thoughts because my body is not constantly sending me signals that I am in danger. It's finally a positive feedback loop.

Given this, I want to break down some of these key nutrients that can impact physical symptoms, because it's important for us to be aware of the correlations between vitamin levels and our mental health. Should you decide to integrate supplementation based on your results, I always recommend working with a provider to get a tailored treatment plan for your body. Supplementation is not a substitution for psychiatric prescriptions and it's best to get a personalized approach for your specific symptoms. I also want to highlight that research continues to evolve and additional studies are recommended to further evaluate the correlations between vitamin levels and the experience of anxiety. Supplementation is certainly not a catchall, but I believe it can be an integral component in treatment that many of us forget, or don't know, to include.

KEY VITAMINS THAT COULD BE IMPACTING YOUR ANXIETY

1. **Vitamin D:** Studies have shown the effectiveness of vitamin D to help manage anxiety, including for those who experience anxious distress in the midst of a depressive episode.[118,119] Symptoms of deficiency include fatigue, bone and back pain, and hair loss.[120] Given that 1 billion people around the world have low vitamin D, with 42 percent of US adults having a deficiency (and even more worrisome, 63 percent of Latinx adults and 82 percent of African American adults), this is one of the most important supplements to pay attention to.[121,122] To improve your vitamin D intake, you should try to be out in the sun for

thirty minutes to three hours, depending on the amount of melanin in your body, and by eating foods rich in vitamin D, including oily fish such as salmon and mackerel.[123,124] If you are lacking in vitamin D, taking a vitamin D supplement can be an essential part of your treatment plan, not only for depression and anxiety symptoms, but also to treat other potential symptoms, including frequent illness/infections. And for you potential mamas who are considering getting pregnant: vitamin D can make a big difference in helping you have a healthy pregnancy, as each 10 nanogram per milliliter increase in preconception vitamin D levels has been associated with a 12 percent lowered risk of miscarriage.[125] Given that supplement level recommendations will vary depending on your demographics as well as the time of year, it's essential to have your bloodwork data as a baseline and to work with a provider for a tailored approach.

2. **Vitamin B:** There are eight groups of nutrients in the vitamin B family. Here's a rundown.

   a. **Vitamin B_{12} (also called cobalamin):** Deficiencies are correlated with paranoia, depression, poor memory, confusion, and fatigue. While about 6 percent of those younger than sixty have a deficiency, about 20 percent of those over sixty aren't getting enough.[126] By eating fish, chicken, eggs, milk, cheese, and fortified breakfast cereals, you can meet the mark. However, given how many of these foods are not vegan-friendly, it's particularly important for vegans to rule out a B_{12} deficiency—especially if you are noticing brain fog and malaise.

   b. **Vitamin B_1 (also known as thiamin):** Most people get these nutrients when they eat whole grains, pork, fish, legumes (such as black beans), nuts, and seeds. However, deficiencies can occur with alcohol dependence, as well as in those living with HIV/AIDS or diabetes, those who are older, and those who have had bariatric surgery. When the body lacks B_1, you can experience memory loss, muscle weakness, and heart problems, among other symptoms, such as loss of appetite.[127]

c. **Vitamin B_2 (also called riboflavin):** This deficiency is rare, especially if you eat eggs, lean meats, low-fat milk, green veggies, and fortified cereals and bread. However, some people can be deficient, including vegetarian athletes (especially those who avoid dairy and eggs), pregnant and breastfeeding people, and vegans. Without enough riboflavin, skin disorders such as sores at the corner of the mouth, cracked lips, hair loss, liver disorders, and difficulties with the reproductive and nervous systems can occur. Long-term deficiency can cause anemia due to a shortage of red blood cells.[128]

d. **Vitamin B_3 (also called niacin):** It's uncommon to lack this nutrient, but it can happen with those who are undernourished, including those with AIDS, alcohol use disorder, anorexia, inflammatory bowel disease, or liver cirrhosis, as well as those who have a diet lacking in iron, riboflavin, or vitamin B_6. When not getting enough, people can experience extreme tiredness, headaches, depression, vomiting, constipation, diarrhea, apathy, memory loss, hallucinations, and aggressive, paranoid, and/or suicidal behavior.[129] If we eat enough poultry, beef, pork, and fish, as well as nuts, legumes, grains, and fortified bread and cereals, our B_3 needs can be met. If not, supplementation is key.

e. **Vitamin B_9 (also known as folate, or folic acid when in synthetic form):** This vitamin is crucial, especially for expecting persons, given that folate deficiency can contribute to babies being born with neural tube defects, such as spina bifida.[130] The CDC recommends that people take 400 micrograms (mcg) of folic acid twelve weeks before becoming pregnant all the way through the first twelve weeks of pregnancy.[131] Of note, females between the ages of fourteen and thirty, African American women, and those with alcohol use disorder are more susceptible to deficiencies. This can lead to megaloblastic anemia, a blood disorder that can cause weakness, difficulty concentrating, fatigue, irritability, heart palpitations, headaches, and shortness of breath. We can get folate in our diet by eating asparagus, brussels sprouts, spinach, oranges, peanuts, kidney beans, and peas.

3. **Magnesium:** While fewer than 2 percent of Americans have a magnesium deficiency, those who are hospitalized, have gastrointestinal distress (such as Crohn's disease or celiac disease), diabetes, or an alcohol use disorder have a greater likelihood of not getting enough.[132] The National Institutes of Health notes that men over the age of seventy, as well as teenagers, may also be at greater risk of magnesium deficiency.[133] Magnesium does everything from regulating nerve and muscle function, blood sugar levels, and blood pressure to helping our body make protein, bone, and DNA. A deficiency in magnesium can lead to a loss of appetite, fatigue, vomiting, and nausea. An extreme deficiency can cause tingling, muscle cramps, an abnormal heart rhythm, and personality changes. We can get magnesium in our diet by eating whole wheat, spinach, quinoa, almonds, cashews, black beans, and my favorite—dark chocolate. The benefits are far-reaching. Magnesium not only has been shown to help women increase their muscle mass and power, it also can help reduce symptoms of depression, prevent migraines, improve sleep, and lessen PMS symptoms.[134] And when it comes to anxiety, a six-week study found that taking 248 milligrams of magnesium per day significantly reduced symptoms of anxiety.[135] A word of caution, though: work with your provider on the dosage, as high intake can cause diarrhea, nausea, and muscle cramping.

4. **L-theanine:** An amino acid found in green and black teas, as well as some mushrooms. One study found that those who drank 200 milligrams of theanine had lower cortisol levels and a lower stress response when completing a challenging task.[136] Given that L-theanine can interact poorly with sedatives, it's important that you consult with a doctor before taking a supplement.

Are you noticing an interesting pattern here? So many of the physical symptoms of vitamin and mineral deficiencies parallel the symptoms of anxiety, depression, ADHD, and even psychosis. We can easily get lost in our heads, wondering, "What the heck is going on with me?" when sometimes there can be an explainable answer sitting in our lab report.

Take this as a call to action: **Get your bloodwork done**.

Yes, everything may come back as normal. At that point, we can integrate other treatment options and tools (and we should anyway). But don't do yourself the disservice of living in the dark about what your body may be trying to tell you. Our bodies give us cues all the time when we're off-kilter, such as when we have frequent migraines, irritable bowel syndrome (IBS), or brain fog. Don't minimize or ignore these signs.

When I invited Suma to get her own bloodwork done, her results were eye-opening. After living with physical anxiety for much of her life and coming to the conclusion that this was "just how it would be," she was shocked to learn that she had a significant vitamin D deficiency, as well as a B_{12} deficiency. She began working with her family doctor to incorporate supplementation and within a month's time, Suma noticed that her physical symptoms of anxiety, including fatigue, low mood, difficulty concentrating, and muscular tension, all began to improve. While Suma and I continued to do the cognitive work to help her with her mindset and behavioral changes, having her physical symptoms abate was incredibly relieving for her. She was able to use her mental energy elsewhere because she was no longer having to constantly monitor and scan for her physical symptoms of distress. She told me three months later that she felt like an entirely different person who finally had her life back.

A NEW WAVE TO RIDE:
Have you gotten your bloodwork done recently? If it's been a while, what stops you from taking that step? What's one thing you can do to take action with this?

THE MIND IS A PART OF THE BODY AND THE BODY IS A PART OF THE MIND

There's a theme here: the brain is not disconnected from the rest of the body. Sometimes we recommend "getting a checkup from the neck up" but honestly, we need a checkup of the entire body to better understand the neck up. That's why I'm such a staunch advocate of things like getting bloodwork done because it gives you a look into what's happening underneath your skin. Westernized care can tend to look at the brain *or* the rest of the body, but they're not two separate entities. They're incredibly connected. The more we look to the entire body to give us meaningful data, the better care we can all have.

It's a two-way street. It's not just that imbalances in our overall chemistry can cause us to feel mentally unhealthy. It's also imbalances in the brain's chemistry that can cause our physical bodies to present symptoms that can mask themselves as purely physical problems. For example, research has shown that when we're under long-standing and/or severe stress, the signaling in the brain can become interrupted or altered, contributing to the experience of not only mental distress but decreased immunity, metabolic and circulatory disruptions, and a host of other unpleasant physical symptoms.[137] Add to this the layers of age, unique genetic history, and life experiences and you can understand why the highway between the brain and body is often congested.

For example, research continues to emerge on the strong connection between gut and brain health. With over 100 trillion bacteria present in our bodies, much of it in the intestinal tract, we are seeing how our gut health impacts our neurological, endocrine, and immune pathways—also known as the gut-brain axis.[138] Given that our gut bacteria make up the hundreds of neurochemicals that the brain uses for things such as regulating our mood and helping our memory, we'd be ignorant if we didn't consider this connection. Specifically, the gut makes up 95 percent of our serotonin supply, which impacts not only our mood but also our gastrointestinal tract.[139] It doesn't seem coincidental that 60 percent of clients with anxiety and/or depression have reported gastrointestinal distress, such as IBS.[140]

Though they are microscopic, changes in the gut microbiome can be significant for our brain health. For example, when we feel stress, it can lead to changes in our gut bacteria, corresponding with the HPA (hypothalamic-pituitary-adrenal) axis in the brain. This then leads to corticotropin-releasing factor (CRF) in the brain to change our intestinal permeability.[141] Layperson's terms: when we experience stress, it can lead to changes in our gut bacteria, which send a signal to the brain that we are under duress, leading to a release of cortisol, which then makes our stomachs more sensitive, and as a result induces feelings of anxiety. This builds on itself as the body continues to detect the ongoing experience of stress.

The good news is that our gut bacteria can also alleviate anxiety and depression. For example, researchers have found that different bacteria strains, such as lactobacillus and bifidobacterium (they sound like Harry Potter spells to me), can reduce the amount of cortisol that circulates when we're stressed. In fact, these bacteria strains have been shown to reverse the HPA axis pattern that induces anxiety.[142] It's important to note that this research was done with mice, but there's a strong plausibility that these findings correspond to what takes place in our human bodies as well. The same study also found that anti-depressants can prevent the amount of cortisol released, which also impacts the gut. This makes sense, given how often clients share that their nausea and gastrointestinal distress subsist after they take an antidepressant.

Now, how can you heal your gut microbiome if you suspect yours may be under attack? Yogurt with active cultures (unheated) and fermented foods (think sauerkraut, miso, kimchi, kombucha, and tempeh) are great ways to get your gut health in high gear. If you're like me and you're a picky eater, prebiotic-rich foods such as raw apples, asparagus, beans, bananas, artichokes, garlic, and onions may help you start to wade in the pool of getting good gut health.[143] It's also important to work with a provider who can recommend the right kind of probiotics for you based on your symptoms and give you instructions for how to take them.

For a quick frame of reference, here are a list of foods that can help alleviate your anxiety—or worsen it. Of course, these foods aren't the recipe for an automatic correlation, but they can certainly contribute to or decrease your anxiety. Why? Some food products can increase inflammation in our bodies, which causes oxidative stress, leading the brain to interpret distress signals that can correspond to anxiety and depression.[144]

That's the thing—the food we put in our bodies can be medicine for the brain, or, at worst, poison. That may sound dramatic, and it's certainly not something to become obsessive about (trust me, it's rare that I go a day without eating some sugar). However, given that we're putting food into our bodies multiple times a day, we have to consider how it impacts our overall health, and especially our brain health. There could be a whole book on this (and certainly there are many—*This Is Your Brain on Food* by Dr. Uma Naidoo is my absolute favorite), but here is a short list to help you get started.[145]

FOODS THAT CAN IMPROVE ANXIETY	FOODS THAT CAN CONTRIBUTE TO ANXIETY
Spinach and other leafy greens (folate helps produce dopamine)	Sugar (sudden blood sugar spikes can make the body feel jittery, irritable, and nervous, while increasing inflammation)
Cashews (full of zinc, which can help reduce stress) and Brazil nuts (high in selenium, which can improve mood by reducing inflammation)	Artificial sweeteners, such as Aspartame, sucralose, and saccharin (shown to contribute to neuropsychiatric problems)
Salmon (packed with protein and omega-3 fatty acids that counteract stress hormones) and oysters (a powerhouse for zinc)	Fried foods, especially when corn oil and soybean oil are used, as is often seen with fast food (increases inflammation)
Turkey (has the amino acid tryptophan, which can help produce serotonin)	Alcohol (causes blood sugar to spike while impacting sleep quality, interfering with serotonin, and also depleting B vitamins)
Avocado (tons of B vitamins)	Caffeine (as a stimulant, it can intensify anxiety and induce panic attacks, while also interfering with sleep)
Dark chocolate (can help suppress cortisol, the stress hormone)	Processed and prepackaged foods (can increase inflammation, negatively impacting the gut microbiome)
Kimchi, miso, and other fermented foods (contain a high amount of probiotics, which help with gut health), as well as yogurt	Gluten (especially for those with an intolerance, anxiety and depressive symptoms can be exacerbated)

Turmeric (contains curcumin, which can help boost serotonin and dopamine)—use it with black pepper to activate!	Dairy (yep, this one is on both sides; it can be inflammatory, increasing adrenaline and decreasing magnesium)
Chamomile (shown to induce feelings of relaxation), peppermint tea (can help relax muscles when tense), and green tea (contains theanine, an amino acid, that can help keep stress at bay)	Sugary drinks and diet and regular sodas (blood sugar spikes can amplify anxious symptoms and these drinks lack fiber)
Eggs (great source of vitamin D and protein)	Foods high in trans fats/hydrogenated oils (think frosting, cake, cookies, etc.), as they contribute to increased inflammation
Berries (vitamin C helps repair damage from stress on our cellular walls) and bananas (high in B vitamins, including folate and B_6, which help produce serotonin)	Foods in cans and plastic containers (may contain BPA, which can impact mood and blood pressure while also impacting fertility)
Oats (a great serotonin booster and it's a complex carbohydrate, satisfying hunger)	Some food additives and food dyes (have shown correlations with anxiety, depression, fatigue, and brain fog)

You don't need to do a total 180 with your diet, but if you can start making some small changes, you might start to see some noticeable differences in your anxiety levels. A breakfast packed with protein, for example, can be a way to stabilize your blood sugar in the morning while helping to improve the functioning of your neurotransmitters in the brain.[146]

And what about approaches such as intermittent fasting? Is it helpful? If you're anxious, I wouldn't recommend it. As it can lower blood sugar, some people notice increases in anxiety, irritability, headaches, and difficulty concentrating, as well as fatigue and sleep interference (so basically most of the symptoms that we see in someone presenting with anxiety).[147] Not to mention, this type of eating often leads to or exacerbates eating disorders. Before you start any big change in how you're eating, it's always recommended that you talk with a doctor or nutritionist to make sure you're getting enough nutrients to fuel you throughout your day.

Ultimately, focusing on putting whole (preferably organic) and unprocessed foods into your body is a great and natural way to combat anxiety. It's not a surefire solution, but it certainly won't make your anxiety worse. I get that this is so much easier said than done. Eating healthy foods comes from a place of privilege. It's expensive to get fresh, organic, and non-prepackaged foods. At the end of the day, it's better to put some food into your body than none. When you can make the choice to eat green instead of plastic wrapped, or raw or steamed instead of fried—great. And if you can't, that's okay too— make do with what you have and do what you can, when you can. It's better to be kind to yourself with how you're feeding your body than to mentally beat yourself up if you're not doing it "perfectly." There's no such thing.

Don't underestimate the importance of staying hydrated as well. Believe it or not, how much water you drink can impact how much you experience anxiety and depression. One study followed three thousand participants and found that those who drank more water were less likely to be anxious, and even less likely to be depressed.[148] Another study noted that dehydrated folks were less calm and more tense compared to those who drank up, who endorsed greater feelings of happiness and contentment.[149] Not to mention, staying well hydrated aids with digestion, particularly with helping the body absorb the nutrients from the food you eat (further supporting that all-important gut-brain axis health).[150]

Part of Suma's treatment plan included taking a look at her diet. I often will do a twenty-four-hour food history with a client to get a snapshot of what they ate in the past day. When we did this, we realized that there were some areas where we could make some changes with Suma's eating plan. For example, she wasn't eating breakfast and would have two cups of coffee on an empty stomach (similar to Mikaela). For lunch she would eat fast food at work and would add a chocolate chip cookie for dessert. In the afternoon, she'd have an energy drink as a pick-me-up. For dinner, she had salmon with green beans and potatoes (a great meal with the omega-3s and greens). Suma was open to making some changes, particularly with her caffeine intake, adding in breakfast, and spending some extra time with meal prepping. Before long, she started to see that she felt less jittery, especially in the morning, when she changed to black tea (coffee to green tea was too big a jump at first) with a high-protein breakfast to help with her blood sugar. She added in more colors of the rainbow, shooting for three a day (such as carrots, strawberries, and spinach), and she started to feel more energized as a result. She also started to have snacks on hand, such as a yogurt or a nut pack, so that she wouldn't get dizzy from getting too hungry. In a matter of weeks, she saw how food changed her mood—and the differences were so noticeable that she felt it was worth the effort to keep eating differently.

AS YOU CONSIDER THIS, I INVITE YOU TO TAKE A LOOK AT YOUR OWN PERSONAL DIET. LET'S START WITH A TWENTY-FOUR-HOUR FOOD LOG. WHAT DID YOU EAT IN THE LAST TWENTY-FOUR HOURS?

_____

_____

_____

_____

_____

GIVEN THIS DATA, WHAT DO YOU MAKE OF HOW YOU'RE EATING ON A DAY-TO-DAY BASIS? WOULD YOU SAY THAT YOUR NUTRITION MAY BE HELPING, HURTING, OR A BIT OF BOTH WHEN IT COMES TO YOUR BRAIN HEALTH?

_____

_____

_____

_____

WHAT ARE SOME POTENTIAL CHANGES YOU'D LIKE TO MAKE TO SEE WHETHER THEY SHIFT YOUR EXPERIENCE OF ANXIETY? THIS MIGHT INCLUDE CUTTING BACK ON CAFFEINE, LIMITING ALCOHOL, ADDING IN MORE FISH OR LEAFY GREENS, OR TRYING TO EAT A HIGH-PROTEIN BREAKFAST MORE OFTEN. LIST WHAT YOU'RE OPEN TO TRYING OVER THE NEXT TWO WEEKS:

1. _____

2. _____

3. _____

4. _____

5. _____

COME BACK TWO WEEKS LATER. DID YOU NOTICE ANY DIFFERENCES IN YOUR MOOD AS YOU MADE THESE CHANGES WITH YOUR NUTRITION?

_____

_____

_____

_____

DON'T UNDERESTIMATE THE POWER OF SLEEP

It's not just about what you eat, though. Given that we spend about 33 percent of our lives asleep, and considering that sleep problems impact more than 50 percent of people living with generalized anxiety disorder, it's worth discussing sleep hygiene and the benefits of getting enough rest.[151,152] Insomnia and anxiety is a bit of a chicken-and-egg situation: it could be that when we're anxious we have trouble falling and staying asleep, and when we're lacking sleep we feel even more anxious. It's the worst kind of biofeedback loop.

One of the best things you can do if you struggle with insomnia is to practice *accepting* it. I know—completely counterintuitive. But what often happens is that we get ourselves so worked up that we're not sleeping that in the process, we get ourselves even more agitated, making it harder to fall asleep. If we practice accepting that we're struggling to sleep—and if we don't get threatened by it—that can often help us relax enough so that we can drift off.

When we're upset about our inability to sleep, it's often tied to a fear that we'll be in pain the next day. You know the feeling—when you can barely keep your eyes open, and it physically hurts to be awake. It's no walk in the park. And yet, it's *survivable*. If we can remember that the pain is temporary and that we can endure discomfort, the insomnia doesn't have to be so threatening. Remind yourself of all the times when you've been able to get through tough days, even on little sleep. It's not ideal, but it's doable. And worst case, if you need to call out with a sick day or cancel a meeting to take a nap—do it! If there's an opportunity to alleviate some pain if you're suffering, don't be a martyr to the cause. Take a break. The point is that the pain of exhaustion does not need to be feared—remind yourself of your resilience. And remember—when you are intentional about lying down and resting (even if you're not actually asleep), that does the body good! This is restorative in itself. If you mentally beat yourself up for not being a good enough sleeper, here are just a few examples of some reframes I used with Suma when she was struggling with insomnia at first:

INITIAL THOUGHT WHEN FRUSTRATED WITH INSOMNIA:	REFRAMED THOUGHT:
"I'm so upset that I can't sleep! What's wrong with me?!"	"I'm noticing that I can't sleep right now. It might not be pleasant but it's okay to be awake right now."
"I'm going to feel miserable tomorrow. I'm going to flunk my test because of this."	"I may not feel great tomorrow but it's just one day. I've gotten through hard days feeling tired before and I've still performed well. Plus, I can take a nap after my test if I need it."
"This is such a waste of time to lie here. This is doing nothing for me, being wide awake."	"Even if I'm not asleep, my body is still getting rest by lying here right now."

If you're like Suma and your anxiety can get the best of your sleeping habits, here are some sleep hygiene tips.[153] Some of them may seem simple enough—but ask yourself, how many of these do you actually follow through with?

- Put your cell phone in another room to charge: if this feels too difficult, at a minimum, put your phone on silent and facedown so that you aren't getting pings and blue lights popping up at two in the morning.
- Listen to sleep stories on the Calm app (who wouldn't want to drift off listening to Harry Styles's voice, after all?).
- Set aside your electronics at least thirty minutes before bedtime.
- Try to go to bed and wake up at the same time each day, including on weekends. This helps to balance your circadian rhythm.

- Keep your bedroom quiet, dark, and cold (between sixty and sixty-seven degrees is ideal).[154]
- Don't have a TV or computer in your bedroom.
- Refrain from large meals before bedtime (hello, heartburn) as well as alcohol (which interferes with your REM cycle multiple nights after you have a drink).[155]
- Stop drinking caffeine at least six hours before bed.[156]
- Get some exercise, just not one to two hours before bed, as this may keep you awake.[157]
- If you can't fall asleep after twenty minutes, get out of bed and do a quiet activity, such as reading, with minimal light exposure. Don't whip out the phone!
- Use your bed only for sleep and sex.
- Reduce fluid intake before bed so you're less likely to need the bathroom in the middle of the night.
- Talk to your provider to see whether melatonin or another sleep aid may be helpful.
- Try using earplugs and/or an eye mask to cancel out noise and light.
- If you do need a nap, keep it short, to no more than twenty minutes. This helps boost alertness without slipping you into deep sleep.[158]

While we're hoping to get seven to nine hours of sleep a night, just like with the foods you put in your body, have compassion for yourself.[159] Beating yourself up mentally for failing to get enough sleep isn't going to help the cause. If you continue to struggle after trying these strategies, I recommend working with a provider who specializes in CBT-I: cognitive behavioral therapy for insomnia. It's also worth doing a medical evaluation, including a sleep study, to rule out any potential diagnoses such as sleep apnea, nightmare disorder, and narcolepsy. If you've been suffering for an extended period of time—if you've been struggling for more than, say, a month—and you're finding that the lack of sleep or feeling of exhaustion is regularly interfering with your waking hours, this may be an indication to get yourself some additional support. You don't have to keep toughing it out.[160]

JUST KEEP SWIMMING . . . WHEN YOU CAN

When we get anxious or depressed, we often want to hunker down and move our bodies as little as possible. When we're immobile at home, this can be a part of an extended freeze-like state that can evolve into a dissociation. It can also feel like a profound physical lethargy that feels all-consuming. While it can temporarily feel comforting to lie as low as possible, we have a wealth of research that advocates for doing the exact opposite. Moving your body—and, no, it doesn't have to be anything vigorous like training for a marathon—can be incredibly helpful for your mental health. Whether it's a gentle yoga practice, walking for twenty minutes, or going for a swim, we know that getting some exercise can make a fundamental difference in the experience of anxiety.

How so? Harvard Health Publishing reports that when you get your heart rate up, this changes your brain chemistry, including the availability of antianxiety neurochemicals, such as serotonin, gamma-aminobutyric acid (GABA), brain-derived neurotrophic factor (BDNF), and endocannabinoids. These can act like natural painkillers that also improve your ability to sleep. Additionally, exercise activates the frontal cortex of the brain, which helps downplay that overly active amygdala that so many of us have. Exercise also has a musculoskeletal impact, relieving muscle tension, which is seen all too often with anxiety. Lastly, exercise often gets our minds off whatever it is that we're feeling anxious about. The power of distraction—especially through exercise—can't be underestimated.[161]

Given that we often dread the physical symptoms that anxiety bears on our bodies, exercising can help us become more comfortable with the sensations of a racing heart, sweating, and feeling out of breath—not too different from how the body can feel during a panic attack. We can reduce our anxiety sensitivity through exercise as we see how survivable these sensations really are. While anxiety can make us feel weak, both physically and mentally, regular exercise helps us see just how strong we are.[162] Almost inevitably, this builds your confidence and comfort with your body. In fact, though not true for everyone, it's been shown that exercise can be just as effective as taking an antidepressant.[163]

I've seen the power of this in my own life. Because my anxiety often shows up physically, I can be the first to sit home on the couch and turn into a little mummy. However, it was when I read Michael Easter's book *The Comfort Crisis* (in one of my mummified states) that I learned about the power of a misogi.[164,165] The idea of a misogi stems from the Japanese Shinto practice of ritual purification by standing under an icy waterfall. It represents the notion of the body being able to handle discomfort in order to tap into what we're truly capable of. It's a physical and psychological exercise where we learn the magnitude of our strength—which anxiety often makes us doubt.

That's when I asked myself what my misogi would be. As someone who couldn't run more than two miles, I felt that running a half-marathon was practically impossible—but *possibly* doable. Now, for some of you that would be a cakewalk. For others it would be way too much. The point is not to compare yourself to anyone else—it's more about setting a physical challenge that is specific to you.

And so, tired of becoming a corpse on the couch, I literally searched on Pinterest "half-marathon training for beginners." Lo and behold, I began running, slowly adding miles over the three months of training. It wasn't easy. I was about the slowest runner on the block, but I put in the time. Eventually the effort paid off. I'll never forget the feeling when I crossed the finish line and ran the 13.1 miles (with some walking involved around miles ten and eleven, let's be real). I remember feeling

shocked by what my body could do. All those years when I underestimated myself and said that I "wasn't a runner"—it was simply untrue.
My body was stronger than I ever realized. And the best part? I've never
had less anxiety than during that training time. Not only was the time
spent exercising a meditative practice in its own way (I loved listening
to music while I ran), my body felt more in balance than it had in years.
While I was skeptical before of how much exercise could really help
with anxiety, this experience made me a believer.

Perhaps this will inspire you to come up with your own misogi. Or
you can shoot for the recommended thirty minutes of exercise, three to
five days a week to help reduce depressive and anxious symptoms. If
your time is limited, even ten to fifteen minutes can make a difference.[166]

If you were to do a misogi, what would yours be?

YOU DO YOU

When I first met Suma, she told me that she felt such pressure to just
do therapy or take medication. She was especially hesitant to take
medication. I totally respected her decision, reminding her that while
it's my job to let clients know all the treatment options available to
them, it's also important they pick self-care and healing strategies that
work for *them*. This is where the incorporation of complementary and
alternative medicine (CAM) practices can be helpful. Many of these
treatments have extensive histories. For example, China developed
traditional Chinese medicine (TCM) in 200 BC. Korea, Japan, India,
and Vietnam also have their own long-standing traditional treatment
interventions as well. While some may be skeptical about these forms
of care, my thought is that if you are making a fully informed decision
and you believe the treatment will help and not harm you, it can be a
useful supplement to conventional medicine.

While some diagnoses may require medication as part of the most
effective treatment plan, as with schizophrenia and bipolar disorder,

for example, there are so many additional supplemental aids that can benefit anyone. We need to expand our view of what can work. Just as how research has shown that therapy is most effective when the client-therapist relationship is strong—regardless of the therapeutic orientation and interventions, the most effective self-care strategies are likely those that feel most congruent for the client.[167] Given that at least more than 38 percent of Americans utilize CAM treatments, with satisfaction with treatments landing at about 71 percent, it's important that we include a whole host of options for healing.[168,169]

Of course, it's worth mentioning that there is the possibility that these additional treatments may not be effective for you. At a minimum, they should never harm you or make your symptoms worse. It's also worth noting that many of these treatments are not always covered by insurance, which is important to consider before you pay for different options. Furthermore, given that some of these treatments may not have as much empirical support, there is the possibility that you don't always see the improvements you're hoping for. However, you just might find that some of these strategies offer their own forms of transformative healing. Whether they help you process a trauma, or you notice a reduction in the physical experience of your anxiety, perhaps it's worth giving some of these additional sources of support a shot if you're open to it.

Here's a list with some ideas to get you started as you consider what you'd like to incorporate into your own treatment. This list is by no means exhaustive. Once again, keep in mind that not all of these modalities have extensive research demonstrating their effectiveness—in fact, some have shown limited support for symptom improvement when clinically tested. However, if a particular addition to treatment works well for you and benefits your overall well-being, then good for you. As you look through this list, circle what has helped you in the past, as well as what you're open to trying. Notice whether you feel any judgment or skepticism pop up as you consider these options. This may mean a particular option might not be the most helpful for you, though it may be effective for someone else.

Acupressure

Acupuncture

Affirmations

Animal therapy

Aquatherapy

Aromatherapy

Art therapy

Astrology

Aura healing

Ayahuasca retreat

Ayurveda

Biofeedback

Body wraps

Breathwork

Cannabis/CBD

Chakra healing

Crystals

Cupping

Dancing

Detoxification

Dream interpretation

Drinking tea

Emotional freedom technique
    (tapping)

Enneagram

Equine-assisted therapy

Eye movement desensitization
    and reprocessing (EMDR)

Family therapy

Feng shui

Float therapy

Forest bathing

Gardening

Going out in nature

Going to the chiropractor

Gratitude practice

Hiking

Homeopathy

Hot bath

Ice bath

Improv/theater

Infrared lighting

IV therapy

Journaling

Laughter therapy

Lymphatic massage

Martial arts

Massage

Meeting with a medium

Meeting with a spiritual leader

Mindfulness exercises

Music therapy

Naturopathy

Nutrition

Pilates

Play therapy

Poetry

Prayer

Progressive muscle relaxation (PMR)
Qigong
Reading books
Reflexology
Reiki
Religious practice
Running
Sand therapy
Sauna/steam room
Self-help books
Sensory deprivation
Sewing/knitting
Sex therapy
Singing
Stretching/foam rolling

Supplements
Support groups
Tai chi
Tantra
Tarot reading
Traditional Chinese medicine (TCM)
Transcranial magnetic stimulation (TMS)
Traveling
Visualization
Walking
Weighted blanket
Weight lifting
Worship
Yoga

Once Suma realized that her healing could include so much more than just traditional talk therapy, her lens for recovery widened greatly. She began doing yoga and loved adding in some peppermint aromatherapy when she felt particularly panicky. Getting a monthly deep-tissue massage was restorative for her, as well as taking the time to connect more deeply with her Hindu faith. She saw that her healing was multidimensional. It was a daily practice that took effort and time. As she saw herself become a grounded human being, she told me that her self-care was worth it. For the first time, she committed to a regular plan of action and she saw the difference. It was undeniable to both of us.

We often want quick fixes for our pain, but investing in a treatment plan that works for you is a process that will pay off gradually, not after the first session. Your own plan of healing will take time.

But what about when the body takes over and it feels like none of your coping strategies are working? Read on.

WHEN A WAVE KNOCKS YOU OUT

If you tend to get panicky—you're not alone. In fact, every year, 11 percent of Americans experience a panic attack at least once.[170] Part of why we can feel panicky is because the vagus nerve, the longest cranial nerve in the body, can get dysregulated and start ricocheting a whole host of unpleasantries in the body, including but not limited to IBS, heartburn, dizziness, tachycardia, seizures, and migraines.[171] The vagus nerve holds tremendous power in our bodies as it toggles back and forth between our fight-flight mode and our parasympathetic mode, which is when we feel more at ease. Feeling anxious can be an indicator that the vagus nerve is not cooperating with us. Thankfully, there are some quick ways that you can start to regulate it. Bookmark this page to turn back to as a quick reference the next time you feel panicky:

- **Use cold water:** A chilled drink on your forehead or a thirty-second cold shower can trigger feelings of relaxation.[172]
- **Sing along with music:** Not only does singing strengthen our breathing muscles and upregulate immunoglobulin A, which improves our immune system, the physical act of singing or humming stimulates the vagus nerve when we exhale.[173]
- **Get a twenty-second hug:** This releases the cuddle hormone, oxytocin, in our bodies and can bring a sense of peace and closeness while increasing our heart rate variability.[174]
- **Breathwork:** By practicing diaphragmatic breathing (where you can feel your belly expanding), the vagus nerve is activated and we have improved oxygen saturation.[175] If you're confused by this or not sure how to practice belly breathing, lie on the floor and put a few books on your stomach. This will help you feel your stomach filling with air, rather than your chest. There are so many great breathwork apps that can help you with this, including Calm, Headspace, Insight Timer, and more.

Whether you're grappling with panic attacks, struggling with insomnia, or wanting to be more intentional about the food you put in your body, I hope this chapter will help inspire you to settle into yourself. Invest the time to understand what's going on beneath your surface (start by getting your bloodwork done!) and then take the steps to actually heal. This won't be a one-and-done resolution. This is a lifetime of daily choices—it's a lifestyle. Living from a place of wellness takes dedication. It's a lot easier to no-show on an appointment than to do the work sometimes. However, when you show up for yourself, you're sending your brain and body a powerful message. You are explicitly saying that you are worth it—that you deserve care.

As Suma came to see, things can get better when you take action. The waves of anxiety will come and go, but you can learn how to ride them. Don't give up on yourself or your body. Give yourself time and gift yourself with options. Your approach to your care can be creative. You may have felt like a prisoner to your anxiety, but don't forget—you also hold the keys that can release you from the pain. Now it's time to pick them up and see which ones work.

A NEW WAVE TO RIDE:

What are some steps that you'd like to take toward your wellness to grow mentally, physically, and emotionally this upcoming week? With sustained effort, how do you think you might feel differently in a month, six months, or a year from now?

CHAPTER TEN

WHEN YOUR SURFBOARD BREAKS

Things started out fairly routine with Sam. They wanted to discuss their recent breakup with a partner. As a queer, nonbinary, white, atheist person, they had been to therapy before and had a positive association with it. They considered this a "tune-up" to process their new relationship status. While they were disappointed that the relationship didn't work out, they weren't distraught. They were simply giving themselves space to reflect and feel. You go, Glen Coco.

But then, things changed. Overnight.

Sam came to their session in tears. I'd seen them upset—but this was next level.

I said, "Sam, what's going on? I can tell something is wrong."

They answered, "I can't believe I'm telling you this . . . but my family home burned down last week."

"What?" I was shocked.

"Yes. A fire blew through town so quickly. The winds were wild. One minute we were told to evacuate and the next we were driving up to see our house in ashes. I just can't believe it."

I responded, "Sam, this is truly awful. I am so, so sorry."

We sat together while they cried. Nowhere to be but here.

Sam eventually said, "This just can't be real. I have so many memories in that house. Christmas Eve dinners. Birthday parties. Getting a puppy and playing with him in the backyard. To know that it's all gone is devastating. I can't accept it."

My heart ached for Sam. While I hadn't lived out their pain directly, I had felt something close. Being a California psychologist, I've had many clients experience the trauma of ravaging fires, and it's hit close to my own childhood home. While my family narrowly escaped having our home burn down by the Thomas fire in 2017, my best friend, also named Lauren, lost her family home that day—on her birthday. I'll never forget hearing her tell me while I sat on a plane, "It's all gone, Lauren. My home is gone." All of our childhood memories flashed before my eyes: building forts in the backyard, playing with Barbie dolls in her playroom, and dressing up for Halloween in July (we always took months to plan out our outfits in advance and still do to this day). When she told me the news, I immediately started crying on the plane. I didn't care that people saw. Her home was gone and there was no getting it back. Even though I keep the memories that happened there, it's haunting to know that the place where they all took place is no longer here. So, when Sam told me this news about their home, I had a sickening sense of how shocked they felt. It was a death of its own kind.

Whenever a tragedy like this occurs is usually when people come in with some toxic positivity phrases. "At least no one died," or "They're just things—things can be replaced." Sure, that's all true. But it's traumatic to have your home, your potential safe haven that you've known and loved for years, torn away in a matter of hours. It's a pretty awful feeling to drive through your neighborhood and not know whether your house will still be standing. I certainly wasn't going to minimize Sam's pain. It was an irreplaceable landmark of their life that disintegrated all in one night.

When tragedies like this happen, I have a name for it: evil popcorn. It's when, for no rhyme or reason, some are saved and some are not. It's this evil popcorn that keeps us up at night—we never know when that kernel might pop. It's enough to send us into a panic if we let ourselves.

Sam got hit with evil popcorn when their home burned down. Maybe you've been hit with it yourself. Sometimes it's being in the wrong place at the wrong time and our worst-case scenario happens. Other times, we know that the pain will be inevitable. Sometimes you see the pop coming and sometimes you don't. It burns your tongue all the same.

The pain can be inevitable; it can be unpredictable. What do we do with that? This book has so far been about learning to ride through the toughest of waves, but, hell, sometimes the wave is just too big for us. Sometimes it breaks us. That's what this chapter is for—when life feels snapped in half. When we've been bitten by the shark and it feels like we've lost our leg (or maybe we actually have), how do we heal?

Here's where to start: get out of your water. Stop forcing yourself to swim. I love Dory from *Finding Nemo*, but she was wrong this time around. Don't "just keep swimming." No—you need to take a break. I'm amazed at how many clients (and non-clients who feel like they don't need therapy) force themselves to keep working into oblivion so that they don't have to sit with the reality of their pain. When anxiety is in the mix, it can feel practically impossible to slow down and make room for our sadness. We'll do anything to avoid looking at our grief. But surprise: no matter how fast or long you try to swim away from your heartache, it's still there, waiting for you. You may as well acknowledge its presence before it makes you. So give yourself grace and step out. You're not strong because you keep forcing yourself to swim—you're strong because you're brave enough to get on dry land when you need it.

Bookmark this chapter if you're grieving right now. Or save it for a rainy day when you get that phone call you never want to get. You don't need to work through this in any particular order. All that I'd recommend is, as you can, settle in with your pain. Rather than turning away from yourself, look at the wound. See the pain for what it is. It's hard to know how to heal if you're not facing it. After all, would you want a doctor to give you stitches if they weren't willing to look at the cut? We have to see our pain so that we can give ourselves what we need to recover.

GIVE YOUR BODY WHAT IT NEEDS

One of the most important ways that we can process our grief is to allow our bodies to physically process what we've lost. Whether we cry, shake, scream, or even get physically sick, we need to let our bodies do what they need to do. Your brain may think it knows best by shutting down any physical display of emotion, but your body knows exactly how to heal if you give it the permission.

This can be incredibly hard to do if you struggle with anxiety. When we're scared, we want to exert control, especially over our bodies. When a situation already feels out of control, it can be even more distressing when we feel like we're at the mercy of our bodies as well. Many of us will try anything to stop our pain from popping up—so much so that we'll have a panic attack to replace it. The more we try to bottle up the tears, the anger, or the physicality of our symptoms, the more they can burst open in the exact ways we were trying to avoid. If we instead give ourselves the grace to experience our emotions fully, the more grounded we actually tend to feel. Shifting your perspective on what your body does in the grieving process is restorative. It's not trying to hurt you. By expressing itself physically, it's trying to heal you. We wouldn't need to fear our bodies if we knew this, because we'd remember that they're working for us, not against us. Your body can be your friend—not your enemy.

Instead, many of us fight ourselves tooth and nail. Some of us even seem to have a magical ability to suck our tears back into our eyes. I've seen many clients do this; they will do anything to avoid crying (they'll change the subject, laugh, drink water, avoid eye contact, etc.). Even in therapy, a place where crying is invited, we stop ourselves from ever shedding a tear if we can help it. And yet, crying is incredibly healing for our bodies. When we cry, we not only are clearing out stress hormones and other toxins from our bodies, we also get a hit of oxytocin and endorphins. This helps ease both physical and emotional pain.[176] That's why when people say that they "just need a good cry," they mean it.

I invite you to welcome the tears. If you feel like you're able to cry at a moment's notice, give yourself permission to express your emotions. You don't need to shame yourself for feeling upset.[177] But if it feels hard for you to access your tears—as it does for many folks with anxiety, as they've gotten good at cutting themselves off from their physicality—try some of these tools.

- Listen to music that brings up sadness, anger, or any other feeling that you'd like to evoke.

- Watch an emotional movie where you resonate with the story (*Marley & Me, A Walk to Remember,* and *The Notebook* do it for me).

- Write in a journal while looking at a picture of something that reminds you of what's upsetting you or what you've lost (while listening to music, to add on an extra layer).

- Sit in your car or go for a drive by yourself—there's just something about that space, especially when, once again, you're listening to music.

- Get past the small talk. Say something that's in your heart and go deeper with someone. Set the jokes aside for a while and share the truth of how you feel.

I realize this may be sounding a bit masochistic at this point but, truly, taking time to emotionally process your loss is paramount. Those feelings are already there inside you and you need to let them out. If you don't, you'll likely feel the sadness manifest as physical sickness. The body wants equilibration when we're in pain. We're not far off from our fellow animals in this regard. The fight-flight-freeze response is ingrained in each of us and when we experience a stressor or a loss, the body wants to react physically in order to seek homeostasis again.

Denying ourselves this instinctual need is a form of personally gifted torture. You don't need to do this to yourself.

Dr. Peter Levine has done some incredible research regarding how our body processes stress, including trauma.[178] His work began when he noticed how animals demonstrate physical spasms and flailing to complete the fight-flight cycle, particularly after they had been stuck in the freeze state.[179] For example, when a polar bear has been in shock, its body will eventually come out of this state by shaking and panting. By doing so, it's discharging stress hormones that otherwise would get trapped in its body. It's a completely normal process that regulates the polar bear after it has been in a state of fear. We don't judge the polar bear for doing what it needs to do.

Now cue our human response. While we too may want to shake, tremor, cry, and physically react, we lock it down when we feel upset. We learn at a young age that we're "babies" or we're "crazy" if we express our distress. We are told that we need to be "brave" and as we grow up, we think we are "being strong" by shutting down any physical response that could cue us or others that we're scared or shaken up. Problematically, when we do this, the stress hormones that are released, regardless of our external reaction, get trapped in our bodies like a Ping-Pong ball. Unable to process them, we start to get headaches, gastrointestinal distress, brain fog, body aches, and exhaustion. Sometimes we feel dissociated, moving through our lives like we're in a haze. We learn to resent the body, even though it has been trying to help us all along. Before long, we feel cut off from it entirely, paying attention to it only when it gives us pains that we can't ignore, such as a panic attack or sickness so severe that it keeps us in bed. In fact, studies have shown that experiencing long-lasting stress (e.g., as a result of ignoring your grief) can lead to an increased risk of developing autoimmune disorders and serious infectious diseases—further justifying why it's so important that we pay attention to our bodies.[180,181]

This is where Levine's method comes in. Rather than stiffening the body, or ignoring it altogether, he invites us to welcome the body's sensations, which he calls somatic experiencing.[182] This can include allowing the body to shake, tremble, and self-regulate as it needs to.[183] If you think this sounds strange, you're right on track. We've been socialized to think that losing control of our bodies is "weird." In fact, the only way this form of movement has been considered mildly socially appropriate is when we dance (but even then, it's when people get themselves "loosened up" with alcohol and still, we love to judge one another from the sidelines).

Embracing your body in all its uncontrollability sounds unnerving if you're not used to it. In fact, you've likely been trained to feel averse toward it, thinking that something is "wrong" if your body doesn't do exactly as you command. It sounds counterintuitive to welcome or even invoke the feeling that the body is out of control. Anxiety tells us that we're "losing it" if we don't have our physical sensations under control. Heaven forbid someone see us shake, cry, or display fear with a cracked voice, cotton mouth, or sweat. But as evidenced by throwing up to rid the body of toxins when we're sick, or shaking during the childbirth process, our bodies have an innate wisdom about what we need. If we're willing to surrender to what it's telling us, we can move through our pain and our process in a much more organic way. It doesn't mean it won't still hurt. We just won't have the added fear or exhaustion of trying to stave off the body's natural (and restorative) healing.

The problem is that we think we know better than our biology. We don't trust ourselves. As a result, we walk away either feeling disconnected or in constant dread of what our bodies might do to us.

What would happen, though, if your body's reactions didn't warrant shame? What if your body could do what it needed to do without your judging it, or the fear that someone else would?

I know with my own phobia, my fear is entirely about losing control of my body and, worse, that other people will be disgusted by me. It boils down to a primal fear of embarrassment. I have to remind myself that others can have compassion if I get sick (even though I may lack it for myself and others, sadly). My body is just trying to look out for me.

Similarly, many of us have a deep-rooted fear of being humiliated and ultimately rejected—whether it's socially, emotionally, or physically. That's why we apologize when we cry in front of others. It's why we won't dance in public or go to a workout class where other people could watch us moving our bodies. We let our kids move their bodies exactly how they want to, but for some reason when we get older, we're not allowed to play in the same way. And what about when someone has uncontrollable movement? We see things like shaking as a sign that we're unwell. We try to hide it from others—even though it's an indicator that the body is trying to restore balance.

If you shame your body or worry that others will think your grief response is "too much" if you have a physical reaction, the toxicity of the trauma or loss will continue to stay trapped inside. Your body needs to work through the loss—not just in your brain. As we've covered before, it's all interconnected. **Your brain doesn't just need to talk it out; your body needs to feel it out.** Here are some helpful ways you can engage in some somatic experiencing. Of course, please be mindful of what feels comfortable and doable for you. Go at a pace that works for your body—respect what you need and what you can do.

- Practice some exercises that allow the body to shake (a ballet barre class is great for this, as well as Tension & Trauma Releasing Exercises [TRE]).[184]
- Literally "Shake It Off" with dance as Taylor Swift recommends.
- Engage in tapping exercises (Emotional Freedom Technique, or EFT).[185]
- Get a massage or do a stretching session.
- Sit in a rocking chair and rock back and forth. Just as babies find the rocking soothing, so do we!
- Do a yoga, Pilates, or other body movement class.
- Go for a run or walk where you're noticing your breath and body parts work together.

Your body has innate wisdom. In our Westernized society, we can get so cut off from that wisdom. It amazes me that in all my years of clinical training, we received extensive information on cognitive interventions and yet rarely covered any body work. Just the other day when I told a fellow psychologist about the power of somatic therapy, she responded with "What's that?" It goes to show how little we in our field have been trained to appreciate the power of the body.

Now, to be fair, somatic experiencing hasn't been studied as extensively as cognitive behavioral therapy. But does that mean we should disregard it if it is bringing healing to folks? Our bodies can tell us just as much as our brains, if we are only willing to listen. So, in the gentlest way, perhaps you can start to lean in and get curious about the messages that your body is trying to tell you. Go slow and get to know the friend, not the enemy, that is your body. Your body knows how to work through your heartaches—if you only allow it.[186]

WHEN YOU NEED TO GET ON DRY LAND

Like I said earlier, there are times when you need to get out of the water entirely. It might be when your pet passes away, when you have a miscarriage, or when you're diagnosed with an illness. We are so encouraged to push through our pain and sometimes, we don't have a choice. But this is where I'd like to suggest that if you do have the space to take a respite—you do it. We often feel like we are weak if we need a time-out. We go to work a week after our divorce finalizes or we stay in school when we're grappling with the aftermath of a parent passing away. But hear this: you don't have to tough it out. If you need to get out of the water, by all means, do it.

Now, I hear you already: "But keeping myself distracted allows me to forget about the pain. It's helping me cope." Is it, though? While you can busy yourself at times, you ultimately have to face the ghost of grief that is lurking in your shadows. There's never a good time for pain. I don't know a single person who says, "Yep, now would be a good time for my sister to pass away. I'm ready." Yeah—said no one ever. You can try to postpone your pain, but trust me, it's going to still be waiting for you. And then there's this . . .

This is probably going to sound weird to you but in some ways, grieving can feel *good*. When we honor what we've lost, we're acknowledging the meaning that has been present in our lives. It's hard to grieve something if it didn't matter to you. And not to say that you should feel guilty if you don't feel upset by a recent loss, but there's a difference between ignoring pain that is clearly there and forcing feelings that weren't there to begin with (which is totally okay, by the way). Ultimately, honoring our grief is a way to honor ourselves. It's a form of self-care. When we acknowledge that our healing process is more important than deadlines at school or work or the comfortability of our friends, we're giving ourselves a powerful message of self-love.

This is something I had to remind Sam of. They were so ready to jump into action with everything that needed to get done after their home burned down. Sam was masking their emotional exhaustion by physically exhausting themselves with an endless list of to-dos. They made it impossible for any emotions to come to the surface because they were so preoccupied with their tasks. Their body was starting to deteriorate, too. Letting go of sleep, eating well, exercise, and just straight up sitting with their sadness, they began experiencing a profound fatigue. Their stomach hurt, their head ached, and their skin became pallid. They looked and felt miserable, but they felt that they had to throw themselves into their work as a way to cope.

I called this out in session one day. "Sam, I'm worried you're not taking care of yourself. I can tell that your body is hurting. I think it's trying to tell you something."

They hesitated. "What will happen if I slow down, though? Won't I only feel worse?"

"You might at first. That sadness and pain may be felt in its entirety. But you won't be expending so much energy trying to fight it off anymore. What do you think your body is trying to tell you?"

I could tell Sam knew. "That I need to sit with it. I need to listen to it."

"What's stopping you from doing this?"

In Sam's case it wasn't that they were afraid of their body's reaction. They just worried that no one would be there to catch them if they fell. Even though they had people offering to help them, Sam was pushing away this support at every turn.

You might notice this about yourself as well. Maybe you don't allow others to help you when you're grieving or suffering because that means you would actually have time to slow down and be still. There would be room for you to feel your feelings—and the idea of that frightens you. But maybe we can start giving ourselves permission to accept assistance from others when it's offered—or better yet, we can ask for it. It's okay to ask for a hand; you're not a burden or an inconvenience if you do. If others don't have the bandwidth, it's on them to assert the boundary. You don't need to put that wall up in advance, though.

Many of us have learned to hate resting and sitting with ourselves because we're afraid of what we might find. We run from our feelings so often, as we're afraid of their power and what the heck they could even be. Many of us sit in a state of well-placed and ever-present anxiety because it buffers any of the sadness, anger, or disappointment that could be simmering below. Even if grief gets loud enough that we actually have to pay attention to it, we feel like we need to move past it as soon as possible. We try to timeline our pain. We tell ourselves we should be "back to normal" as soon as possible. Heaven forbid we inconvenience someone or make another person feel uncomfortable by our grief.

You need your self-care more than ever when you're in a season of sadness, though. Putting a countdown clock on how much time you have to rest isn't going to help. Take the time that you need. When you start should-ing on yourself by saying, "I should be over this by now," or

"I shouldn't be so upset by this," you're only shaming yourself further. You feel how you feel. And that's okay. After all, if a friend were grieving, would you say to them, "It's been six months. Time's up. Move on." Probably not. So why are you putting these harsh parameters on yourself? You're not impressive because you got through your grief the fastest. Sorry to tell you, but there's no trophy for speediest griever. That's a record you don't want to hold.

We've all collectively grieved in our own ways over the last few years. Whether we lost loved ones to COVID-19, didn't get to walk at our graduation ceremony, or had to quit our jobs to stay home and care for our family, we all had our own unique losses. I can't tell you how many times I would hear clients minimize their pain. They would say, "I shouldn't be sad. Others have it so much worse than me." Sure, there is always someone that has it "worse" than you. But are you sad? Are you disappointed? That's all that's required to get yourself a golden ticket to the gates of grief. No one wants to go there, but there aren't VIP passes that warrant which rides you get to go on. You don't need to compare your grief to others. It is what it is. There's no one who can take away how you feel—and that includes how you treat yourself.

I try to model this for my clients. I'll never hide what I'm going through if it's going to potentially impact how I show up in session. It's important to me that my clients know that I'm a real human being, just like they are. As I would hope they could set boundaries if they needed a break, I want to show that for them as well.

I'm reminded of when I had to take some time off when I almost lost Mochi. He hadn't even turned five yet and he had been gradually and unexplainably losing weight for months. Things took a turn when he was coming out of anesthesia after getting an ultrasound. We found out Mochi was in sepsis and the vet told me he had a 50 percent chance of making it. The vet told us that she would call us during the night if Mochi didn't survive. I've never been so afraid for the phone to ring.

Thankfully, the phone didn't ring that night, but Mochi went through a harrowing few weeks to recover (he even had a feeding tube).

I can honestly tell you that I've never been so upset in my life. I remember sobbing for days on end. I even ordered a stuffed-animal Siamese cat off Amazon just so that I'd have something to hold. I saved his tufts of fur that he left around the house (yep, I was that upset). Even though he didn't die, I was still wracked with the shock and anguish of almost losing him. During that time, there was no way that I could be present for my clients. I could have tried to push past and ignore the pain, but it would have been a disservice to my clients and to myself. I had two priorities during that time: to help Mochi heal and to make room for my own emotional pain. By the grace of God (and an incredible vet staff with modern medicine), Mochi recovered. I'll always remember how, when we finally got to take him home, he picked up his head and started purring the loudest we'd ever heard. He was just as excited as we were that he finally got to go home.

As I'm writing about this on the anniversary of this ordeal, I'm keenly aware of how traumatic this was for me. Mochi may as well be my child and I'd do anything for him. I'd never been so distraught before and the weight of my distress took even me by surprise. Now, I could have shamed myself in the grieving process—telling myself to get over it. Some of you may be thinking, "Wow, Lauren. He's just a cat." I could have turned bitter: swearing to myself that getting a cat was a mistake because almost losing him hurt so bad, and therefore I would never do it again. I could have resented how much all of his medical bills cost. I could have tried to swallow my tears and keep a stiff upper lip.

But I look at grief another way. I see it as a reflection of how deeply you love something or someone. When the tears flooded out uncontrollably, it simply told me how much I loved this little being with all of my heart. Sure, he's a cat. But he's *my* cat and he's given me more love and comfort than just about any other living, breathing being (sorry, Greg—although you're pretty great, too). I know this is true for many of you who have had pets as well. They've given you care and companionship unlike any other. That relationship is indescribable. When we lose them (or almost lose them), it's okay to feel the magnitude of it. It's not insignificant.

So whatever you may be going through—or will go through at some point—take the time that you need. Whether you've lost a pet, a job, a home, a marriage, a baby—don't diminish it any way. It was yours for a precious piece of time. Not having it anymore can be profound. There's no point in judging how you grieve, either. Allow yourself to honor what's been exceptional for you. It was so important that I helped Sam hold this. The home that was beloved to them would no longer be what it was. There was no going back to it, even if it was rebuilt. That's a hurt that's not worth ignoring. We took the time in our sessions to reflect on the significance of that home—how they came to understand their gender identity and fall in love for the first time in that house. They drifted away from their parents and got close to them again in that house. Like in the Miranda Lambert song, it was a house that built Sam.

As you process your own grief, see whether you can start to let people in. You don't have to keep your pain in like some shameful secret. You don't have to silently sob or pretend you're not crying with one of those dumb "it's the onions" jokes. Let yourself wail. Curl up into a ball. The people who love you want to be there for you. Do what you need to do to restore yourself—even if that means doing nothing but crying, reflecting, and sitting in one place. There's no right way to grieve. No one should be pressuring you—including you yourself—about how to proceed.

LET A LIFEGUARD IN

Sometimes we feel like we have to bear our suffering alone. You don't. While it's good to take time on your own to reflect, you're not a burden to others if you are in pain. You don't need to go into a play-by-play of what you've gone through (unless you want to), as some research has even suggested this may not be helpful.[187] What is helpful is to allow others to support you, whether it's with meals, conversations, or just sitting together and watching a movie. You don't need to be embarrassed by your pain or minimize it in any way to make someone else feel more comfortable. You're a human with a beating heart. Sometimes that heart bleeds when we've lost something extraordinary. That's okay.

You don't need to feel guilty about asking for what you need. Sometimes people can get flooded by their own anxiety and may retreat when you need them the most—it's not because they don't care about you. It's more likely that they're afraid of doing or saying the wrong thing when you're already in distress. That's why you don't need to be shy about being explicit with how they can help. Give them meal requests. Ask them to help you out with your kids. Even though lifeguards are trained to look for people who are silently drowning, it doesn't hurt to put a hand up and say exactly what you need if you're able.

At the same time, if you're reading this and you're wanting to support someone who is grieving, don't be shy about jumping in. It's better to make a misstep (such as not saying exactly the right thing or overstaying your welcome) than to not be there at all. The most important thing to remember is that your presence alone is what is needed most. You can't replace what has been lost but you can buffer the edges of the new gap.

And as much as we can help each other out, sometimes the lifeguard we need to let in the most is ourselves. Acknowledge the change that has taken place in your life. Reflect on what you've experienced and how it's changed you—for better, for worse, and without judgment. Begin to develop a narrative of what you've gone through. It's helpful to jot down your memories of the person you've lost, the experience you've had, or what the journey has meant to you. Note the feelings that are attached—are you shocked, confused, disappointed, or angry? Make room for those feelings to bubble up without judgment. As you process your experience, it doesn't mean you "find the reason" for why things happened as they did. As is often the case with grief or trauma, there's no good reason. We can learn and grow through the experience, but part of the processing is sitting with the reality that sometimes that evil popcorn struck in your life and it just plain sucks.

One of the best things you can do as you process your loss is to honor what has happened. While you may engage in a public ritual, such as a funeral, 80 percent of people also engage in a private ritual to reflect on what has happened.[188] This can be impactful if you're seeking closure over a breakup, a job change, or a friendship ending. I often do this with clients, including with Sam. They decided that they wanted to frame a picture of their house and put it up in their new room. This was a way for them to remember the memories that were encapsulated in their family home. They didn't want to forget, and the photo was a way to remind them of that home's significance. It wasn't a memory to be buried.

You can engage in your own ritual. It can be something you do one time, daily, or on an anniversary. This can be a healthy way to process your pain, rather than push it away. Having a ritual can also integrate the loss into your daily lived experience more often—it doesn't have to feel like a distant memory that grows more and more faint. Here are a few ways that you can incorporate a grieving ritual into your life:

- Wear something that represents the loss (a necklace, a ring, etc.).
- Get a tattoo that symbolizes the relationship.
- Have a place that you visit that brings back important memories relating to the loss.
- Put up a picture that reminds you of the relationship, either in a frame, on your phone, or on your computer screen.
- Carry something with you that makes you feel more connected to the person.
- Write a letter to the person or experience that you've lost.
- Light a candle while you reflect or meditate on what's now missing.
- Listen to a song that reminds you of what's changed.

A NEW WAVE TO RIDE:
Is there someone in your life who is grieving and you would like to support? Is there someone you could let into your life to support you? How can you honor the losses you've experienced with more intentionality?

WHEN YOU'RE AFRAID OF THE WAVE THAT'S COMING

Grief is inevitable. Part of what gives so many of us anxiety about grief is that we don't always know when or from where it's coming. This unpredictability is what shakes us to our core. And because we doubt our ability to cope, we worry that we're just one wave away from utter collapse. I've seen so many clients struggle with this form of anticipatory anxiety—they're petrified of losing something they hold dear—so much so that sometimes they never want to get in the water to begin with. Why get a pet when you know it will die? Why fall in love when you know that relationship will someday end? Why try for a baby when so many things could go wrong? The potential for heartbreak can be enough that we practically stop our hearts from beating altogether. We stop living our fullest lives because we're so afraid of the crack that could shatter our glass.

This anticipatory anxiety can quickly lead to separation anxiety. People often think this looks like the four-year-old clinging to their mom's pants when they're getting dropped off at preschool, but let me tell you, I've seen many grown adults metaphorically clinging to the pants of their loved ones. In fact, about 6.6 percent of the adult population experience separation anxiety disorder, with 77.5 percent reporting that the initial onset came on during adulthood.[189] So as much as we may think that it's just little kids who have a hard time saying goodbye to Mommy when it's time to go to school, there's actually a lot of us—especially those of us who are prone to anxiety—who struggle with saying goodbye (or the possibility that we would have to say goodbye).

It's understandable that we fear the day when we will no longer have our loved ones beside us. We're hardwired to be deeply connected social creatures. Not having our beloved with us is a thought that dismantles many of us. But there's a difference between occasionally worrying about the potential day when we'll lose someone we hold dear, and agonizing all the time about when that day will come.

Before we go on, let's just take a moment to assess how intense the separation anxiety may be for you.[190,191] Note how many of these hold true for you.

1. _____ You dread having to say goodbye to your loved ones and put off having to part ways.

2. _____ You avoid getting into fights with loved ones because you're afraid it could be the last time you see them.

3. _____ You check in with your loved ones daily to make sure they are safe and you feel guilty if you forget to reach out. You may even monitor their behavior and their health to ensure they're not putting themselves in potential danger.

4. _____ The holidays can be especially nostalgic and bittersweet, where you wonder whether this will be the "last time" that you're all together.

5. _____ You often have visions or nightmares about the worst-case scenario happening to your loved ones.

6. _____ Even though you may need alone time, you push yourself to be with others because you feel a pressure that this could be your last chance to have quality time together.

7. _____ You feel like you will never be okay again once your loved one passes away or if they were to leave you.

8. _____ You have trouble leaving your home or another place where your loved one lives. You'd rather be with them than go somewhere new by yourself or to meet new people.

9. _____ You often have somatic symptoms (headaches, nausea, panic symptoms) when a goodbye is coming up or happening.

10. _____ Every time the phone rings you worry that something bad has happened.

If a lot of this is hitting home for you, you're not alone. I would argue that our generation has seen an uptick in separation anxiety. Why? Because we have so much unpredictability in our lives. Things have changed—drastically. No one and nowhere feels safe. Many of us now refuse to go to movie theaters, shopping malls, or concerts because we're so afraid of what might happen. The grim reality is that we never know when our loved ones could be ripped from us.

Even though our world is considered safer than it was even in the 1990s (which as a true Millennial I consider the golden era of Spice Girls and Disney Channel original movies), we don't trust our security in this world.[192] In fact, while half of all Americans report that they feel unsafe at some point *every single day*, more than 75 percent of younger Americans between the ages of twenty-five and thirty-four note that they feel nervous about their safety on a daily basis. That means that only 25 percent of young adults feel safe as they move about their lives. Fifty percent of us won't use a rideshare service because we feel it's dangerous. We don't trust others and we don't even feel safe in our own homes. Forty-two percent of us, when home alone, feel unprotected—myself included.[193]

I would argue that September 11 was a significant event that shaped our sense of security in the world for Millennials and Generation Z, just as the COVID-19 crisis will likely shape Generation Alpha. On a fateful fall day, what began as a seemingly normal Tuesday morning turned into one of the most epic tragedies of our time. We witnessed a massive amount of death and destruction on our television screens while we ate our Cheerios. It changed everything. All of a sudden, nowhere felt safe anymore. Anywhere and anyone could be a target. This unpredictability—and this exceedingly public display of trauma—changed our sense of stability forevermore. And even though Generation Z might not have as much conscious recollection of the experience, they've now grown up in a world where their parents had to internalize such brutal terrorism.

I've had so many clients report that 9/11 was a transformative event that changed how they viewed the world. It was the first time their anxiety really kicked into high gear. We lost our sense of control (which was never exactly there to begin with). Even now, I see clients go into panic attacks when they hear that Kim Jong-un is testing missiles again. Folks feel chaos when they hear that Putin continues to invade Ukraine. In the United States, it's rare that we go a week without hearing of some mass shooting—the only questions are how close was it this time and how many people died or were wounded. The unpredictability of violence is enough to unnerve us all. So it makes sense that we've got more anticipatory anxiety than before—we never know whether *this* will be the last time we're hugging our loved ones.

When it comes to loss, especially unexpected and tragic loss, it's practically impossible to know when that day will come. This is where we have a choice to make, though—and this is where your empowerment lies. We can choose to constantly fight the idea that we *might* lose our loved ones tragically or experience a profound loss. Or, we can choose to accept the reality that anything is possible.

This doesn't mean that we operate devoid of logic. While anything can happen, we can keep in mind that the likelihood of our worst fears coming true is actually fairly low. For example, you're more likely to die from an accidental opioid overdose than a car crash. The odds of dying from gun violence is, on average, 0.0045 percent. And dying from being a passenger on an airplane? According to the National Safety Council, there were too few deaths in 2020 to even calculate the odds.[194,195]

At the same time, we have to acknowledge that we live in a world with disease, natural disasters, and heartbreak. One in six will die from heart disease and one in seven will die from cancer. A statistic that floored me was learning that in 2020, one in twelve people died from COVID-19.[196] In addition, in 2021 the Emergency Events Database reported that there were 432 natural disasters throughout the world, impacting 101.8 million people, with 10,492 people dying.[197] And the reality that we will all, at some point, lose someone we love dearly? One hundred percent. Even though it's inevitable, it can be hard to accept nonetheless.

When you've been hardwired to see your anxiety as a protective factor that might magically prevent this pain, leaning into this notion of acceptance is beyond counterintuitive. In some ways it feels like giving up—like we don't care enough if we don't worry ourselves silly. But here's the thing: your anxiety will not be the saving grace that protects you from your pain. That pain will come (or not) regardless of your anxiety. Believing that your anxiety is serving you is a false premise. It's only exacerbating your distress.

This begs the question: What would happen if you gave your anxiety up? I know it's not that simple, as it often feels automatic and uncontrollable. But what if you stopped seeing your worrying as something that was protecting you? What if, instead, you believed that you had the ability to cope? That your pain was not something to be feared but rather accepted as a part of the human condition?

We live in a broken world. Bad things do happen—but they don't *always* happen, as much as the news would like you to think they do. We're inundated by negative events and it can seem like the majority rather than the minority of our experiences. It's not by happenstance that as the news cycle has become twenty-four hours and the scrolls on our phones have become bottomless, our mental health has deteriorated. People can create anything on social media and say it's truth. We're fed a specific algorithm that knows exactly how to cater to our specific fears. I see it all the time as my community on TikTok tells me that my posts on separation anxiety, anxious attachment, and high-functioning anxiety hit a little too close to home. And as we scroll, we're physiologically short-circuited, as we're often fighting with both people we know and strangers as we attempt to distinguish between fact and fiction.

This is different than for previous generations who got their news from the morning paper and the nightly news. Now we have a firehouse of information—all of which has become more graphic, inflammatory, and polarized. It's addicting to stay constantly plugged in as it feeds our anxiety beast. It temporarily feels good to bathe ourselves in information. It feels relieving to know that we're not missing anything. This checking behavior ultimately intensifies our anxiety, though. In fact, a survey done by Digital Third Coast found that during the pandemic, 68 percent of people said the news left them feeling more anxious, and about 66 percent of respondents said that they felt overwhelmed and burned-out by the news.[198]

This is once again where our empowerment can come in. Just because the news is constantly there, you don't have to consume it. It doesn't mean you're an ignorant citizen of the world or that you're avoiding reality if you don't watch or read about current events for hours a day. You can still stay aware without soaking up so much toxicity constantly. When you've integrated acceptance, you know that tragedy exists. You acknowledge that fact. You're not constantly on the lookout for the possibility of loss because you know it's a reality. However, you also don't drown yourself in distressing news because you know that you can handle pain and discomfort if and when you have to.

Instead of doubting your ability to endure (and hence the need for your ever-present anxiety), you can begin trusting that you can cope with whatever comes. You can handle pain. It's not pleasant—not by any means. But you also trust that you can find a way through.

If you've never experienced loss, you may be wondering how one simply trusts that they will survive through pain. That is one of the side effects of grief: you learn that even when your worst nightmares come true, the darkest night does not last forever.

Sam saw this firsthand. They told me how they used to worry all the time about their home burning down, especially since it was on a hillside and they'd had more and more close calls through the years. They used to lose sleep worrying about what it would be like someday if their home went up in flames. They thought they would never be able to get through it.

And then, one day their worst fear came true. It actually happened. While Sam was shattered by the loss of their home, they also told me over the next several months that the reality of the pain was not nearly as intense as what they had imagined. While they were heartbroken, they were learning how to pick up the pieces. Were they a changed person? Absolutely. But through their tragedy they also saw how much other people cared about them, in a way they had never known before. They had an opportunity to evaluate what really mattered to them moving forward in their new beginning. They never would have wished to have lived through such devastation, but alas . . . here they were—living and breathing through it one day at a time.

And I have to say this because I know you're thinking it. But what if I don't make it? What if it is too much? What if I die of the pain?

This goes against everything in our paradigm of anti-death but here goes: *so be it*. Death happens sometimes. It's usually not what we want but it is a part of life. Just as we have to accept pain, we have to accept death. This is *so* hard to sit with. In a world where surviving is assumed to be the ideal, some of us can even force others to keep living—whether or not it's what they want for themselves. Even when a person is ready to pass, we don't always want to allow it because we don't want to sit with the stillness of our own pain. Like I said, anxiety can make us selfish sometimes.

Ask yourself what scares you so much about death. Is it the unknown? The permanence of it? That it is an ending before you feel ready? The injustice of it? These are all plausible fears. None of which can prevent a final outcome that may just be what it is. I don't mean for this to sound callous. I'm just naming the reality of what our anxiety is murmuring to many of us every single day. We fear death so much that we ruin our living years worrying about what could be.

I realize that you may be thinking I'm cruel at this point. Why on earth would I be bringing all this up when I know it hurts? Because even just reading about death, including your death and the death of your loved ones, or the possibility of "emotional death," is a form of exposure therapy. It's a form of processing and preparing. Avoiding the ultimate reality of death only enhances our fears surrounding it.

This is where empowered acceptance is warranted. When we can acknowledge this universal truth about death, we can learn to live that much more fully. We no longer have to live in fear of the possibility of dying because we've accepted that it's not a possibility but a reality. There is power in owning this truth rather than running away from it.

Your empowerment lies in how you choose to live your life. Death will be waiting for you either way, as will the death of experiences, people, and seasons of life that you hold dear. Don't let the impending goodbyes stop you from the hellos and all that comes in between. Goodbyes wouldn't matter so much if we didn't allow ourselves to love one another so deeply. Don't stop yourself from leaning in because you're afraid of the fallout that will be waiting on the other side.

COMING BACK STRONGER THAN EVER AFTER A WIPEOUT

There are a lot of things in life that can break us for a time. But like starfish, we can grow back from our wounds. One of the best ways to not let our anxiety win is to not allow it to keep us down. While we need to process our pain, we also can seek justice and restoration after a tragedy has occurred. Otherwise, if we only accept but don't take action, those same tragedies can keep repeating. If we keep seeing our homes, like Sam's, burn down but don't do anything about climate change, more homes will be affected. If we keep watching discrimination occur repeatedly but never take steps to stop this, it will continue—perhaps becoming more and more subtle, but just as harmful. We're not always going to agree on how this should all be handled, but the point is that we care enough to do something about it. Healing can come on a collective level when we see that our suffering is not just about remedying our own pain. It's about doing what we can to prevent unnecessary pain for others as well.

Anxiety can make us feel like we need to do it all—right now. We feel that if we're not doing everything in our power all the time to rectify every tragedy, we're failing. We're not. Do what you can, when you can. Sometimes one of the best things we can do is simply to learn and talk about these things so that we're building an awareness for how we can improve our communities. It's the avoidance—when we want to put our heads in the sand—that is ultimately damaging for us all.

I saw Sam jump into action after their home burned down. Ultimately, it was tremendously healing for them. They began getting involved in climate change awareness programs and they spoke at their local community meetings to discuss how the government could help prevent hillside fires in the future. They became fascinated by the various ways that we can protect our planet and even did some presentations at nearby schools to share how students could combat climate change. Sam wrote letters to their local and state representatives. The experience of the fire, while they wished it had never happened, changed them *for good*.

They told me one day, "I never knew that I could care about something so much. I would never wish this experience on anyone, but going through this has opened my eyes to just how dire our situation is."

I shared with Sam how inspiring their passion was. It was contagious. It even motivated me to do my own research on climate change. I started eating less red meat and talking with Greg about how we could save more energy in our home. It reminded me of how change can have powerful ripple effects that touch lives even beyond what we're aware of.

It's true, you can't solve a problem if you don't realize it's a problem in the first place. Accept what is. Face it head-on. After all, you can't ride a wave if you don't know how big it is. And then, once you're strong enough to paddle, get on the freaking board and ride that wave. Own the water. Your voice has more power than you think. Anxious or not, use what you've got. Help us turn these tides of tragedy in the direction that we all need to go. We need you more than ever—and I'd venture to guess that you need it for yourself, too.

CHAPTER ELEVEN

GETTING BACK OUT THERE AFTER A WIPEOUT

Most therapists either love or hate couples therapy. I happen to love it. It's a whole different ball game when you have three people in the room (the couple and the therapist, though sometimes more if it's a polyamorous relationship). Typically there is one partner who is more inclined to do the work. The other one is along for the ride. While I love when couples come for preventative reasons to benefit the overall health of their relationship, many couples wait until they're at their wit's end. Couples therapy is their Hail Mary pass. At its most morbid level, couples therapy can feel more like hospice care than restorative work. Sometimes it's more a matter of a relationship dying peacefully than ending tragically without closure.

Why does this matter, given that this is a book about anxiety? Well, if ever there was a place for anxiety to rear its ugly head, it's in a relationship. Whether it's spurred by anxious attachment, obsessive thoughts about the relationship, or an inability to commit, there are all kinds of ways that anxiety can rock a relationship. And that's when everything may be going generally well. When things really turn sour, our relationships can wreck us completely. As we just finished the chapter on grief and what to do when we've been tossed and turned in our waters, we'll now cover how you can get yourself back out there again when someone has broken your heart or your world has been flipped on its head. While you may be swearing off love if someone has done you wrong, you can't let that damage stop you from connecting ever again. And even if you're not in a relationship at present (and/or don't want to be), this information still applies to friendships, colleagues, and family dynamics. We've all been hurt by someone at some point in our lives. We've all been burned at some point. This is about creating your comeback story so that you don't continue to stay on the outskirts of your own life.

Given this preface, I was interested to see how it would go when Grace and Ryan came onto the Zoom screen together. I could feel her trepidation and his hesitation before we started. Grace was a straight, Buddhist, Chinese, cisgender woman dating Ryan, a straight, Christian, white, cisgender man. They had been together for ten years and there was a pivotal question lingering in the air: Would they get engaged? Grace wanted an answer and Ryan was skeptical to give one. I was not there to be the tiebreaker. My job, as with all my clients, was to help them come to their own conclusions. After all, while I'm there to support my clients in swimming in their waters, I'm not meant to be the lifeguard who can save their, or any, relationship. Ultimately, it's each couple who must want it for themselves.

It wasn't that they hadn't been trying to figure things out before they got to me. They were facing some major hurdles where it was getting impossible for them to find a middle path. With some instances, no matter the couple, there's not much compromising. What are some examples of these nonnegotiables? For starters: babies. You can't have half of one. Ryan wanted many and Grace didn't want one. And then there's marriage. You're wed or you're not. Grace wanted the ring and Ryan was hesitant to get on one knee. Lastly: where to live. You can't live in Boise and Los Angeles. You typically have to pick one. Ryan wanted to be in a city and Grace wanted a rural area. In the end, someone wins, and someone loses. The best thing they had in their corner was that they each wanted the relationship to work out. They loved each other deeply and had ten years invested in a partnership that mattered a great deal to each of them. Perhaps that was part of the problem, though. Their love for each other (as well as a great sex life) was complicating some clear disagreements that showed no signs of resolving.

That's why I'm going to tell you right now that this isn't a story about how their fairy-tale dreams came true with each other. There was a happy ending, but perhaps not in the way you'd expect.

I worked with Grace and Ryan for quite some time. To their credit, they were both brutally honest about what they wanted in their future. We did an extensive dive into their values so that they could each make an informed decision about how the relationship fit into their lives and their futures. Ryan was clear about the fact that he wanted a family more than anything. He envisioned a bustling household that put *Cheaper by the Dozen* to shame. Grace was the opposite. As an introvert, she hoped for a quiet life with Ryan, traveling when they could and working on fixer-upper houses as a hobby together. She didn't see a pack of kidlets as part of her story. She wanted Ryan to be hers and for him to declare this relationship as his own. She didn't see a point in continuing the relationship if marriage wasn't a part of the equation.

That's where I saw Grace take control of her situation. She was empowered as she accepted the reality of the relationship. And be prepared—I expect you to probably have a strong reaction to this: she set an ultimatum. Yes, you read that right. Grace said from the start that she would give therapy six months. If Ryan was still unsure about marrying her at that point, she was out. He would either know by then or he wouldn't—either way it was an answer.

Now this is where some of you may be saying, "But if you really love them, you'll wait forever." "Why do you need a ring to prove that your partner loves you?" "If they're not ready yet, then it's never going to work out. You're a fool to stick around this long anyway." "What if they only propose because they don't want to lose you and then they secretly resent you?" Or my favorite, "This is sounding too hard. Relationships that are meant to be should come easier."

Well, if you've ever lived with a partner with anxiety or you've lived with it yourself, then you know that few things ever come that easy. It's in the nature of the anxious brain to hem and haw, to doubt, and to be indecisive. We always need *just a little more time*. It's not that we don't love whom we are with. For some of us with anxiety, it can feel really hard to take that next step into the unknown. It's scary to jump in the pool, even if we know we want to be in the water. This is where Grace and Ryan had been sitting for ages. They each hoped that the other would make the jump ahead. Ryan hoped Grace would change her mind about having kids. Grace hoped that Ryan would love her enough that he'd be willing to forgo having a family. Both were too anxious before therapy to fully broach the situation.

This is where something like a time ultimatum can really come in handy. Boiled down, ultimatums are simply boundaries that are clearly elucidated. If you are honest about what you want and what your values are, that's not something to be apologetic or feel guilty about. We often shame people, especially women, for giving ultimatums (ahem, boundaries), when really, they're just naming exactly what they want and by when. Ultimatums are about respecting your time—and the time of the person you're with. Rather than leading you to slowly build resentment if your wishes do not come to fruition, ultimatums make sure there are no surprises if and when you need to leave to find your values fulfilled elsewhere. You're giving people ample opportunities to work with you—or not—when you're giving an ultimatum (boundaries, once again for the judgers in the back). That's the thing—just because you're asking for something from someone, it doesn't mean they have to give it to you. In fact, they can make their own choice and decline the offer. Everyone has informed consent in the process.

Timelines can be incredibly effective for helping you assess whether to stay or go in just about any situation. After all, it can be hard to gauge whether it's just a short spell of dissatisfaction or you've got a more long-standing problem on your hands. For example, if six months go by and you're still miserable at your job—that's a clue that it may be time to be brave enough to look for a new opportunity. If you've had a conflict with a family member and you've given them feedback on how you'd like to see the situation resolved, and they don't take you up on making those changes, that's powerful data. If you want to see a partner get sober and six months later they're still getting drunk and/or high— you've got some answers, my friend. Of course, you can keep waiting and waiting—that's your prerogative. But if you've told someone what your expectations are and they still don't adjust to benefit the health of the relationship, and then you *still* stick around, the only person you may be letting down is yourself.

The thing about ultimatums is that they will give you the answers that you've been waiting for. But you have to be ready to not always like the answer that you get. You will get data through the process— information that is irrefutable. And that's the thing: data is data—you can't fight it and you can't ignore it. You can keep making concessions but at some point, you have to face the truth of what you've been given.

Ryan gave Grace data when the six months came up. He still hadn't proposed—or expressed interest in plans to do so. Grace knew at that point what she needed to do.

She started, "I've been thinking a lot."

We all waited. There was no need for prompting.

She continued, "As much as it pains me to say it, I think we should end this."

Ryan startled. Even though he sensed her distancing, it was a whole other thing to hear her words aloud. Eventually he asked, "Are you sure? Can't we wait just a *little* longer?"

With a resigned sigh, Grace responded: "We've waited long enough, Ryan. You know I love you so much. But the reality is that we want different things. I know how badly you want to have a kid. I have to be honest with myself that it's not what I want. And we need to be honest with each other that we're just not going to get there."

"But I can't lose you, Grace. You're everything to me. You're really going to let this go?"

Grace replied, "I know this is so painful, Ryan. Trust me, it's breaking my heart just as much as yours. But I really believe you'll thank me for this someday. You deserve to be with someone who is going to be on the same page with you. And I deserve that, too."

I could see Grace shaking. She'd just said the hardest words she'd probably ever have to say. She was letting go of a relationship she loved for the sake of her own values that were yet to be fulfilled. It was honorable—but brutal.

I was so proud of her for owning her truth and not continuing to wait for Ryan to come around. She had waited long enough and she was true to the ultimatum she set. Even though Grace was devastated in the moment, we all knew that she was doing this out of respect for herself and for Ryan. It wasn't the easy choice—it was the brave one.

They both entered a stage of grief at that point. We continued to work together to process what had happened in the ten years leading up to this moment and how they would peacefully part ways moving forward. We explored how anxiety had been such a cornerstone in their relationship. With Grace's anxious attachment, she was afraid she'd never find another partner and had hoped that Ryan would change his mind. She had unfairly told herself that if she was "enough," he would forgo his values, particularly having children, because she would be "worth it." As we learned through our conversations, it wasn't that she wasn't amazing. It was that Ryan's devotion to his dream of becoming a father was too great. Ultimately, Grace couldn't fault him for this. She also couldn't lie to herself or to him about having children. As much as he wanted them—she didn't. As we discussed it, she felt relieved in being able to own this truth. She no longer had to placate him in hopes of moving the relationship forward.

We also learned how Ryan's own anxiety got in the way. Being the people-pleaser that he was, he was so afraid of upsetting Grace by expressing how deeply he wanted to become a dad. He had let it slide for years, also hoping that somewhere along the way, Grace would change her mind about becoming a mom. He was afraid of the conflict that would come if they really got into the reasons why they hadn't gotten engaged yet. Everything changed, though, when that six-month timer on the clock was set. Everything could finally come up to the surface. They were holding themselves accountable to the relationship and to themselves.

Unfortunately, neither of them liked what came up. They each had to admit to the other that their future didn't include each other. They owed too much to themselves to sacrifice their deepest wishes for another person. It wasn't that they didn't love each other—it's just that they loved their personal values more. This wasn't a selfish choice—it was an act of authenticity that spared them from continued years of pain. I think the only thing they may have regretted was that it took ten years of anxiety to figure this out. They each had kept waiting and waiting for a change to come. As they saw, as is the case when it comes to the consistency of values, it never did.

Perhaps this is something for you to get curious about in your own life. What are you waiting . . . and waiting on right now? Is there something you're desperately hoping will change but at the same time, you're not doing much about it? Perhaps this is where your own ultimatum can come in handy. Give yourself a deadline. Let's play this out:

WHAT'S A CHANGE OR STEP THAT YOU MAY NEED TO TAKE THAT YOU'VE BEEN PUTTING OFF?

_____

_____

_____

IF YOU WERE TO GIVE YOURSELF A TIMELINE TO MAKE THIS CHANGE, WHAT DATE WOULD YOU SET? (TWO WEEKS, THREE MONTHS, SIX MONTHS, A YEAR?)

_____

_____

_____

This is where you can get really honest with yourself. Here are some examples:

- If I'm still hating my job in three months, I'm going to start applying to other positions.
- If they're still not ready to move in together when my lease is up, it's time for me to end this relationship.
- If I'm still feeling the itch to move to a new city in six months, I'm going to take steps to change locations.
- If I'm still miserable at this school at the end of the semester, I'm going to change my situation and apply to other programs.

WHAT'S YOUR ULTIMATUM (#BOUNDARY) THAT YOU NEED TO SET FOR YOURSELF? ("IF THIS DOESN'T CHANGE BY [X DATE], THEN I'M GOING TO [INSERT ACTION HERE].")

_____

_____

_____

The key is that you clearly communicate these expectations with others. If you're dissatisfied with the current standing of a relationship or situation, it's on you to express what you're hoping to see change. Tell your family if they're supporting you with school that you may be transferring. Let your roommate know that you're considering other living arrangements before you bail. People can't read your mind. It's unfair to put parameters in place without outlining them first to the people in your life who will be impacted the most.

Ultimately, you don't need to continue waiting for your life to happen to you. You also don't need to stay in a situation where you're utterly miserable. Even though anxiety may want you to feel weak and deferential, that's not a script that you need to adhere to. You can write your own script and create the conclusion that best suits you. That's not selfish or inconsiderate. You're being honest with yourself and everyone else around you about what actually matters to you. No apologies necessary.

WHEN IT'S TIME TO GET BACK INTO THE WATER

This chapter isn't about the initial crash of heartbreak. It's about how we can pick ourselves back up again, even when we feel jaded and resentful after a loss. If we're not careful, the anxiety of getting hurt again can make us feel like we never want to try again.

We've all seen this pop up in our lives in various ways. We swear off dating after someone cheats on us, feeling like we can never trust anyone again. We refuse to get another dog because it ripped our hearts out when our loving pet died. We promise to never get close with another friend because they could abandon us, backstab us, or drop the ball like the last one did. The more we write others off, the farther and farther we get from allowing ourselves to vulnerably connect.

Now, sometimes, we need to sit on our shore for a while. We need to reflect on what has happened to us before we jump back in the water. While there's no set timeline for how long you should take it easy, remember to listen to your body's cues. If you find yourself crying on a first date or wanting to talk the entire time about how someone did you dirty when you're meeting someone new, that may be a clue that more of a time-out is needed. Grace and Ryan sat together for two months in couples therapy after they broke up. After being in each other's lives for ten years, they each felt that they couldn't be ripped away from each other overnight. The breakup was hard enough as it was. They held each other through that pain before gradually and then fully parting ways.

Eventually, though, there comes a time when you feel courageous enough to dip your toe back in your water. You may need to give yourself a nudge—after all, sometimes it's hard to feel fully ready to let our hearts be loved after a loss. We have to remind ourselves that it's not just anxiety that coincides with a fresh start. There can be passion and excitement, too. If we've been holding ourselves back for too long, we can forget what it feels like to deeply connect with another person, creature, or experience. We forget how it feels to be kissed, to have a pet greet us at the door, or to visit a new country for the first time. We forget how to lose ourselves in play and wonder. Our curiosity is quelled when we write off the value of our vulnerability in new beginnings. We lose ourselves when we're not ready to get lost in the possibilities.

I'd say it's one of the greatest tragedies when a person has surrendered their soul for the safety that comes in the form of anxiety. It's one of the lies our fear would love for us to believe: it's better to never put yourself out there so that you never risk getting hurt. But then you also never risk falling deeply in love or deeply connecting again, either.

It's worth asking yourself: Where are you sitting presently? Are you sitting on your own shoreline right now, watching the waves of your life go by? Or are you in your water, letting yourself ride through the highs and lows that come with each wave? Are you giving yourself a chance to feel it all, even if it feels scary sometimes? Or are you making your own excuses for why now is not a good time to go for a swim?

Insider secret: there's never a good time (just as it wasn't a good time for Jacob either when he called off his wedding). But there's never a good time for loss, and there's often not a good time for new beginnings. When you have anxiety, a new start can be the scariest thing. The great unknown (though it could be truly great) can be more intimidating than a mediocre reality.

This is how I see anxiety being a fake lifeguard that makes you believe it has your back. It will have you believe the ocean is only meant for people who already know how to handle riptides. It tells you that rookies curious about just dipping a toe in the water are not allowed—including you. You internalize that your anxiety must really care about you to protect you from pain in this way. Oddly enough, though, if we all sat on our shores and avoided our lives, as anxiety would like us to do, we wouldn't even need lifeguards because no one would actually ever be in the water. Don't let anxiety manipulate you into believing that you're not worthy or ready for your life. You deserve to enjoy the ride as much as anyone else.

Even as you read this, you may be trying to talk yourself out of your own new beginning. We convince ourselves that we're not ready for romance right now, that this is not the time to change careers or have a kid, or that it's better to postpone that move for next year. That's what Ryan and Grace had been doing for eight of the ten years they were together, when they told themselves it wasn't the right time to get engaged . . . or to break up. Eventually something had to change because the pain of purgatory became too great.

If it hasn't become clear at this point, let me revisit it. *You can handle pain.* You can handle the sting of a job change. You can handle the bite of a broken relationship. You can live with the loss of what you hold dear if it's going to move you toward something that's a better fit. Grace and Ryan sat with the pain and it ultimately benefited them greatly. When they were brave enough to sit with the sorrow, they found peace, and dare I say relief, on the other side.

It's not just about knowing that you can handle pain, though. You also need to know that you can handle joy. So many of us rob ourselves of truly living a life of fulfillment because we feel we don't deserve to be happy or we're too afraid to find out what it actually is that will bring us meaning. Or we think even if we do find happiness, it will never last—so what's the point of having it in the first place? We tell ourselves to settle for what we have because this is "as good as it gets." We feel that it's safer to stick with the status quo so we continue chugging along in our discontent because it's what we know best. For many of us, joy is an unknown box that we're too afraid to open.

I'm not saying to make a change in your life just because. And I'm also not saying that you should expect to be happy all the time. If you fall for this narrative that joy means you're thriving 100 percent of the time, you're constantly going to be cycling out of relationships and jobs as soon as the honeymoon phase ends. You'll peace out the moment there's conflict, boredom, or dissatisfaction. That's not what I'm talking about when I'm referencing this pursuit of unabashed joy. What I'm referring to is how in alignment you are presently. Are you living out the values that matter to you? Are you with someone who sees a similar path ahead or are you hoping and praying that someday you'll get lucky and they'll change their mind on a nonnegotiable, like Grace and Ryan were? Are you absolutely miserable with the work that you do—and have been for years—but you tell yourself this is just how it is going to be? You don't have to settle. And you don't have to keep waiting.

If you have the power to change your situation, even if only by 1 percent, and it will move you that much closer to the values that you want in your life, do it. Giving yourself the chance to find happiness will almost always outweigh the regret of never hoping for better. When you forsake your values for a complacent life, that's not acceptance—that's apathy. There's a difference.

A NEW WAVE TO RIDE:

ASK YOURSELF: WHAT NEEDS TO CHANGE—IF ANYTHING—TO FEEL MORE CONTENT IN YOUR LIFE?

_____

_____

_____

_____

_____

HOW IS YOUR ANXIETY TELLING YOU THAT IT'S NOT A GOOD IDEA TO MAKE A CHANGE? OR THAT YOU'RE NOT READY? OR THAT IT'S NOT WORTH IT?

_____

_____

_____

GIVEN THIS DATA, WHAT DO YOU CHOOSE TO DO MOVING AHEAD?

_____

_____

_____

Let's be clear on this, because I know you might be wondering how to tell the difference between when you need to make a change and when you don't. There's a distinction between boredom and actively feeling unhappy and unaligned. It's normal for all relationships and seasons of life to feel stagnant at times. That's okay. Not everything in life needs to be riveting. We're so used to a harried pace that we've forgotten what it's like to not be constantly stimulated. Stillness is not a bad thing. But stillness is not the same thing as perpetual sacrifice. If you are continually giving up on the values that feel most precious in your life, and you believe you'll have regret if you don't live in alignment with those values, that's your cue that a change may be in order.

That's the thing—I actually believe Grace and Ryan could have been amazing together if their values were on the same page when it came to having kids. They were very compatible and loved being in each other's company. The ultimate problem wasn't their anxiety in the relationship—I believe they could have worked through it and gone on to have a great relationship together. It was that there was an uncompromisable situation on the table that couldn't be sacrificed for either of them—in this case, they couldn't get on the same page about having kids. I admired them both for owning that truth in the end. By accepting the short-term pain of ending the relationship, they were empowered in choosing a relationship that was ultimately a better fit for their lifelong plans. I have a feeling that they both will find the people who are ready to walk alongside them when the time comes.

THESE ARE YOUR WATERS—SO OWN THEM

Looking back, it could have been very easy for Grace and Ryan to resent their situation. They could have each said that their ten years together was a waste of time. I never heard either of them utter those words, though. They both learned a lot through that relationship and had it not been for their partnership, neither would have realized just how poignant their values actually were.

This is where each of us has a choice. We can choose to resent, fear, or accept where we find ourselves. There are so many elements in our lives that are utterly out of our control—our age, our ethnicity, our parents, our ability status, where we are born, and, to a degree, what we look like. Even our experience with anxiety can feel like it is out of our control when our bodies decide to wreak havoc on us.

You can hate the hand that you've been dealt. You can curse the gods and envy those around you who seem to have it easier. This won't alleviate your pain—it will only deepen it. You can also choose to live in perpetual fear of your situation. Worrying that it's only a matter of time until everyone leaves you, you lose everything, and your life falls apart, you can wait by the minute to watch for any signs of unraveling. This is when you're mentally treading in your waters, never trusting what might happen if you'd lie back and float.

Or you can accept the reality of your situation. You can acknowledge what is and what could be. You can face the possibilities with the facts that are in front of you. You can hold both the pain and the joy of your life together—because neither exist without the other in many facets. Ending one relationship allows for a new one to begin. Letting go of one experience makes space for a better one to begin. The pain of goodbye allows for the vulnerable joy that comes with each hello.

Where are you sitting presently? Are you angry about the situation you've found yourself in? Are you constantly scared to be in your situation? Or are you embracing a perspective of empowered acceptance? Be honest with yourself as you consider these examples and how they may map onto your own life:

THE SITUATION	RESENTING	FEARING	EMPOWERED ACCEPTANCE
You're dating someone and it isn't progressing, even though you've been together two years.	You secretly hate that your partner isn't ready to move in together but you're unwilling to have a conversation about it.	You're afraid to say how you actually feel because you're worried that you'll scare them off.	You share what you want moving forward. You give yourself a deadline for progress to happen and if the relationship doesn't move forward by that time, you consider other options. You explain all this clearly to your partner.
You're unhappy with how much you're being paid at your job.	You seethe internally at work and you complain every day to anyone who will listen about how much you hate your setup.	You're petrified to ask your boss for a raise because you're worried you'll sound ungrateful. You don't want to get in trouble for hoping for more.	You have a conversation with your boss about what you feel would be fair compensation. If they're not able to meet you at a reasonable amount that you're okay with, you decide to seek other opportunities.

THE SITUATION	RESENTING	FEARING	EMPOWERED ACCEPTANCE
You feel like your friend is taking advantage of your relationship.	You constantly talk smack about your friend with other friends but you never actually share your frustrations with the person who's bugging you.	You're terrified of losing the friendship so you keep your grievances to yourself. After all, you don't want them to reject you if you speak up.	You share your concerns with your friend and offer them feedback about how they're making you feel. If they're unwilling to acknowledge your perspective and/or make changes, you begin investing your time in other relationships.
Your parent frequently upsets you by saying cruel and passive-aggressive comments about you.	You believe that your situation will never improve and over time, you find yourself hating your parent. Even when something good happens with them, you can't see it anymore.	While they continue to hurt you, you're scared to share how your parent's comments are making you feel. They hold the power in the relationship and you don't want to disrespect them.	You have a conversation with your parent to let them know how their behavior is impacting you. If they are unwilling to see how they are affecting you and shift how they treat you, you learn to set appropriate boundaries to protect your well-being.

Your perspective is your power. In all these situations—and so many others—you can't always control the dynamic that you find yourself in. You can't make people behave in particular ways and there are certainly broader decisions and world events that go far beyond our purview (ahem, here's looking at you, COVID-19). But you do get to decide how you respond. You can loathe. You can complain. It probably won't make you feel any better. You can live in a petrified state, waiting for the possibility of further collapse. Or you can activate empowered acceptance. You can see a situation for what it fully is—and decide how you will respond in turn. It's hard for anxiety to keep ricocheting in your life when you are the one who ultimately decides what you do moving forward.

Sometimes all we have is our mindset. Sometimes everything else can be robbed from us and we can feel like our future is forced upon us. There are real and tangible effects of the uncontrollable tidal waves that hit each of our shores. And while we need to grieve when these storms come to pass, we also do not have to let those waves stop us from continuing to live our lives with a sense of bravery for the future.

This doesn't mean we push aside the pain and the fear that we feel. We can lean in fully to our emotions *and* make room for the good that is still happening in our lives. We can still hold space for hope. It's the dialectic. Our aching can be held with our awing. Like Sam did, we can mourn the loss of a home and see how strong the community is that comes to rally around us. In Grace's case, she was shattered by the loss of an incredible relationship and saw that there was a better fit waiting for her once she said goodbye to Ryan.

Our generation has learned to live in a perpetual state of fear and anger. We're mad about what we see happening in the world and it scares us so bad that we'll either endure the same fate or that it will only continue. Our response has been to isolate, pull back, and resent the predicament we've found ourselves in. This isn't solving anything. We can instead acknowledge our situation for what it is and choose to take steps forward that feel in alignment with the values we hold dear. It may not change the world overnight, but it will change how we feel about ourselves and our future.

You're not broken if you feel afraid. We all do sometimes. If you know what you truly value, and you're committed to living out those values, the powerful urgency of fear doesn't have to pull you out any longer. The reality is that there will never be a good time for you to take a big leap of faith. There will always be an excuse. But do you want your life to be dictated by excuses and postponements or by messy purposefulness? Your life does not need to be curated perfection. Contrary to what Pinterest and Instagram would like you to believe, life is incredibly sticky and no one knows what they're doing all the time. We figure it out as we go.

I'm trying to get into the water too—even though I feel scared sometimes (lol more like every day). Even during this writing process, I've given myself every excuse for why now is not the right time to try to have a baby. Some might say that publishing a book and publishing a human at the same time may not go hand in hand. There's so much unpredictability when it comes to parenting. You could get pregnant the first month you start trying or it could take a very long time. You can have a miscarriage—or multiple. You could have a baby who needs more time and resources than you may have planned for. And so it goes as we enter the unknown. As someone who has tried to plan their life practically to the minute, I'd be lying if I said it hasn't been unnerving entering this season of my life.

Before I talk myself out of it, though, and bargain for another month to postpone my plans, I come back to my own empowered acceptance. I know what I value. I want to build a family—especially with Greg. I know he'll make the most incredible dad and I can hardly wait to see that happen. If I continued to delay, I would be forgoing a long-standing love for something that I know matters immensely to me—all for the temporary alleviation of a potentially inconvenient schedule. Not everything in life is about seeking comfort or the avoidance of unease. I come back to it over and over again: *it's about values induction, not pain reduction.*

I don't have to buy into the narrative that women can't have incredible careers *and* be parents at the same time. Both can coexist. If I allowed myself to indulge, there would always be an excuse for why "now" isn't a good time. That's anxiety, people-pleasing, and perfectionism talking. I know what I want, and I remember deeply in my bones: somehow, in some way, it will all be okay. It will be worth it, one way or another. Anxiety will be along for the ride, but I'm the one calling this shot about becoming a mom.

I get how scary it feels to enter the unknown. It's safer to sit on the shores of our lives and tell ourselves, "Maybe someday." We'll get a new job next year. We'll move eventually. But what I'm learning is that there is never a good time. The timing will never be perfect. You just have to go for it and live in the goop of unpredictability. It's a tall order if you're someone who has lived with anxiety, like I and so many of my clients have. But it's an order that you're ready to fill. If you don't trust yourself yet, I hope you'll trust me when I tell you that you can do it. I should know—I've seen client after client pursue their values before they were ready or when it was incredibly uncomfortable. I've never had any of them express regret for making the brave choice.

As you step forward, I want you to know that you are more than your anxiety. It does not have to define your life. You are not an "anxious person." You are a person who feels anxiety. It is not your identity. Your anxiety doesn't need to stop you from embracing your life fully. Ask yourself what you would do with yourself if fear weren't a part of the equation. *Now do that.* Anxiety does not need to be the excuse anymore.

No matter what your anxiety makes you want to do, whether it's to flee or freeze or postpone, challenge yourself to have an opposite response. You can't control when the anxiety sprouts, but you do get to decide what you do with it. Perhaps it's time to see your fear as simply data rather than as a sole determinant of your life's outcomes.

So, step into your water. I know something has been stirring in you as you've been reading this book. You know what you need to do. You know what conversation you need to have—what choice you need to make. So do it. You're never going to feel fully ready—neither did Grace when she decided to set an ultimatum and when she later told Ryan that the relationship needed to end. Accept the situation as it is—including the fear that you have surrounding it. You don't need to change it or make the fear go away. All that you need to do is take a step forward. This is your empowered action. This is where your power lies—and, not coincidentally, where your joy, your purpose, and your values also lie. I think you owe it to yourself to see that through. You never know what could be waiting on the other side. Don't you think it's time to find out?

CONCLUSION

YOU'RE DOING IT ALREADY

If there's one thing I've learned when it comes to anxiety, it's this: we never give ourselves enough credit for getting through it. As much as people scoff at the "worried well" or the "worrywarts" of the world, anxiety—no matter why you have it—is really freaking tough. It's an exhausting mental battle that we have to show up for. It'd be much easier to run away, and yet, in our own little and big ways, we continue to face our lives. Even with anxiety tearing down the door and trying to drag us down, we've still found a way to get ourselves to this point. It may not feel like it, but we've come a long way.

Are you acknowledging all that you've done to get this far? Are you taking a moment to recognize just how amazing it is that you're doing what you're doing? If you haven't told yourself, hear it from me: I'm inspired by you. I sometimes struggle to get through the day myself, and it's not lost on me just how hard you're working to get yourself here. I hope you can see the bravery that you're living out.

You might be diminishing yourself as you read this. "You're telling me to be proud of myself for brushing my hair today and ordering my groceries online? You're saying I'm winning because I got through my shifts at work this week, even though I'm at a job that makes me feel like I'm a loser compared to everyone else I went to school with?"

Yes, I am. This isn't about comparing your progress to someone else's. You faced your life in your own way today. Bravery is not measured in the magnitude of the event—it's there whether you did the big thing or the small thing, whether you spoke to a crowd of two thousand people or spoke to a stranger on the bus. Both show bravery defined. Anyone who tries to put a metric on bravery has their insecurity on flex.

I know it would probably feel better if we didn't need to feel brave in the first place. If only life would be a breeze and we could be the carefree, happy-go-lucky person we're often comparing ourselves to. Ah, to be chiller. But that's not you. It's not me. Anxiety might be our personal plight but don't forget—that person you're envious of has their own crosses to bear. We all have to stockpile some bravery every now and then—it just looks different for each of us.

As I'm writing these parting words, I'm reminded of the continual ebb and flow of anxiety in my own life. Some days the waves are calm, other days bring a torrent of tidal waves. When I started this book, the seas were fairly still in my life. My anxiety was well managed, and I was coping effectively. I hadn't had a panic attack in two years.

And then . . . as happens in life—the biggest wave of my life thus far hit me.

I found out I was pregnant.

And before I knew it, the empty shores became filled with deep waves of worry that I hadn't seen before. And yes—I had the "typical" worries that many expecting moms have. Would the baby be all right? Would I be a "good" mother? Would I be able to make it all work?

But my anxious brain—the brain that no one seems to talk about publicly—went haywire. With my phobia of vomit still here, each day was a flurry of fear. Would I throw up while giving a keynote speech? What if I got sick during a session with a client? Would people judge me? What if I embarrassed myself? I'm not proud to admit how much these thoughts occupied my mind. But so it is with anxiety. It takes you over like a rip current, and even with your best intentions to swim out, sometimes you get sucked in nonetheless.

And that's when my husband reminded me, while I was having a FaceTime breakdown: "Lauren, I just want you to know, you are being so brave."

I quickly answered, "No I'm not! What if I can't handle all this? What if I can't do it?"

Greg responded, "But you *are* doing it. You are facing it. You're *even more* brave because of how hard this is for you."

I stilled. He was right. I was being brave.

Dare I say: I was being a badass. I wasn't letting the anxiety win. Even though I knew it would be scary and uncomfortable, I *chose* this.

Through all the panic attacks, shaking, relentless ruminating, and checking behaviors—I was doing it. I was still here, getting through each day. It may not have been a pretty picture and I could shame myself for not handling my anxiety "better." But the fact of the matter is this: I am facing my fear. I have to—and that is the choice I am bravely making. If that isn't working through anxiety, I don't know what is.

And sure enough, when I did in fact get sick, I saw how I survived through it. It wasn't comfortable, and I'm in no rush to do it again, but it became clear that my fear of the possibility of throwing up was much worse than the actual reality. Exposure therapy at its best.

I don't know what the future will hold. I'm only nine weeks pregnant as I write this, and I know that I have many waves to still ride through. Some may knock the wind out of me. But I will still keep facing forward. Wave after wave, I choose bravery.

I hope you will choose your bravery, too. Some days you may resent that you need to be brave and some days you may wonder what small crevice inside of you will hold your last stockpile of it. But your bravery is there, just as much as, if not more than, the anxiety that also lies within. Both coexist. As we face our fears, we can see our ultimate strength.

And if you feel like you haven't chosen bravery? I'd rethink that.

Saying no to plans, taking time to rest when we are pressured to always do more, and lying low can also be brave. Being still enough to sit with your thoughts, rather than run yourself ragged into busyness, is brave. In my case, if I had chosen to not have a child, that would have been a brave decision as well. When you say no it doesn't mean you're making that choice out of fear. There can be just as much power in refraining.

Sometimes our fear does win, though. We all have operated out of anxiety and when that happens, the best thing we can do is bravely love ourselves, even if we feel frustrated toward ourselves at the same time. When you feel like you have failed yourself, decide to give yourself compassion rather than shame. If you've been hiding away from yourself, now is the time to be extra kind. You are not going to find your bravery by mentally beating yourself up. Maybe you have been running away today, but that doesn't mean that tomorrow, this next hour—this next minute—can't bring a different choice for you. Just because you may have lived from a place of fear doesn't mean you're destined to always live in the shadow of your pain.

Anytime you show up with an intention, whether that be a mindful yes or no, you are living out your bravery. When *you* make the choice—and not your anxiety—you are riding the wave rather than the wave riding you. And as you do, you may notice your anxiety swell in a whole new way, just as I'm actively experiencing. But at the same time, you'll also see your bravery grow bigger. And it doesn't matter that the bravery feels forced or automatic. Use what you have. Honor that it showed up in the first place.

As that bravery buoys you, remember that you have what you need within you. I hope that you'll have a Greg in your life to remind you of your bravery when you can't see it. But whether or not someone is there to whisper in your ear, know this: *You are strong.* You are brave. You can swim. You can tread. Heck, you can dog-paddle if you have to. You can face this wave that's coming toward you. If you're willing to trust yourself, you'll find that you can lie back and actually enjoy the water around you. Inhale deep, put your legs up, and let your bravery be the breath that brings you to the surface.

THE BEST WAY TO FEEL BETTER

If there's an antidote to your anxiety, it's to care about something greater than yourself. We all have the power to create a trend that evolves into lasting change. You may not be able to champion all causes—but ask yourself: Where do you see injustices in the world? What keeps you up at night? What breaks your heart when you do watch the news? And this: What things are you currently witnessing in our world that if left unchanged you fear will only get worse? These are your cues.

We need to go beyond ourselves. Our anxiety keeps us so small, making us feel like we only have the attention span to keep ourselves alive. But you'd be surprised what can happen in your life when you get brave enough to look up and look out. Once we become willing to hold the pain of our peers, and the people we don't know but still have empathy for, we realize how much we impact one another. We may not be able to resolve one another's tragedies, and we certainly can't prevent every wound, but just knowing that we—and others—are trying to make the world a better place is the salve we all need. After all, wouldn't it be nice to know that someone cares about you? That you matter? That people want the best for you? It goes both ways. When you are brave enough to lean into loving others, the world will open up to you in a whole new way. You will find community with people who challenge you, comfort you, and encourage you. In a time when we feel more alone than ever, we need that collective healing where we show that we care about more than ourselves.

Giving back is one of the best ways to experience more joy in your life. In fact, one study found that 93 percent of people who volunteered over the past year felt happier as a result. That's not all. Eighty-nine percent had an expanded worldview, 88 percent had increased self-esteem,

85 percent developed friendships through volunteering, 79 percent had less stress, 78 percent felt greater control over their health and well-being, and 75 percent felt physically healthier.[199] It feels good to be a part of something that's bigger than yourself. In all the times that I've volunteered, I've never heard someone say, "Well, that was a waste of time." Not once. I know you probably have plenty of things to do, but if there's something to put on your self-care plate, it's service to others—especially with a cause that you care about. Your lack of anxiety will thank you for it.

Because you are 42 percent more likely to achieve your goals if you write them down, I'd love for you to jot down first what you care about, and second, what you can do about it.[200] How can you put this into action in the coming year?

WHAT ARE SOME CAUSES THAT YOU CARE ABOUT? IF YOU'RE STUMPED, WHAT'S SOMETHING THAT MAKES YOU UPSET OR YOU WISH YOU COULD CHANGE ABOUT THE WORLD?

HOW CAN YOU PUT THIS INTO ACTION? WHAT ORGANIZATION(S) COULD YOU SUPPORT OR HOW COULD YOU SERVE THIS CAUSE?

MY HOPE FOR THE GENERATIONS TO COME

As I get ready to take my own action by raising a little human this year (whom I can't wait to meet!), I'm struck by what I hope lies ahead for this *next* generation. I'm fully aware of all the anxiety we've inherited and how easy it would be to pass it right along to those coming after us. I don't think any kid needs much of an education to see how hard the human experience can be. After all, no one chooses to be born, and yet we have to carry the load each day.

My wish is that in all this heavy lifting, we each make it a little (or a lot) lighter for one another. In a world that's mired in pain and tragedy, I want to intentionally be that parent—that person—who brings a laugh, offers a hug, and is willing to simply sit alongside. Rather than teach our children to succeed and achieve, I hope we send a message to simply love one another for the people we are, not for the things that we do.

No matter how old we are, I hope we remember that we each need to be held (both by ourselves and emotionally by others). Rather than run away when it gets tough, we need to comfort one another when our day is rocked with another dose of unsettling news. Even though it can be so easy to stare into the abyss of our own pain (as our anxiety would like us to do), I believe we can each make a different choice to pour out our compassion toward others, not just toward ourselves. The more we're willing to connect, the more we can collectively heal.

With each generation, I see us getting closer and closer to becoming the loving, empathetic people we are meant to be. We are socially built—we are not meant to endure this life alone. As our care for one another grows, I see our anxiety and our self-interest dying in turn. This doesn't mean we're letting go of who we are—we're instead expanding our definition of what is possible.

I come back to a concept that I learned from one of my favorite authors, Reverend Dr. Jacqui Lewis, in her book, *Fierce Love*. She writes about the Zulu term *ubuntu*, meaning, "I am because of who we all are." As I think of this, I can't wait to see how my son will be shaped by the people around him, and in turn how he will shape their lives. As I watch him giggle, play, and cry without any self-judgment—and watch people respond to him—I want to encourage him to keep engaging unabashedly like that for the rest of his life. I hope he never outgrows it. More than anything, I hope his anxiety never tells him to hold himself back from being the person he wants to become. I wholeheartedly hope the same for you.

May we never lose our childlike ability to smile at someone, even if it's a stranger. Let's not forget how to strike up a conversation and truly connect. Certainly, let's not hide our tears just because we're socialized as adults that crying is indecent. Deep down, we're all just kids wanting to laugh, cry, and connect our way through life. Simply put: we need one another.

We may have been and, yes, we may now be Generation Anxiety. But this isn't a predetermined fate for our future. I see a different path ahead. The world will keep handing us its challenges, but as we face them, let's choose something different. We may have a tough road ahead, but I take comfort in knowing that we can at least be a GENERATION TOGETHER.

ACKNOWLEDGMENTS

Writing *Generation Anxiety* has been a dream come true and I'm still pinching myself that this book is on the shelves. I'm beyond grateful for the people who believed in the vision of this book from the start. That begins with Leigh Eisenman, my incredible agent. You saw what this book could be and your belief in this work grounded me every step of the way. There's no one else I'd want to go on this adventure with. Let's have a SusieCakes date soon, yes?

My editor, Soyolmaa Lkhagvadorj—you have been the perfect person to partner with. I trust you fully, and your open heart and mind have been exactly what this book needed. I don't believe too many things in this life are meant to be, but meeting you certainly was.

There have been so many folks at Abrams who have been tremendous. Thank you to Danielle Youngsmith for designing such a beautiful cover that perfectly embodies what the book is all about. Jane Elias, I'm so grateful for your copyediting skills. You polished the book to a whole new level of shine while still retaining my voice. I'm in awe of your talent. David Chesanow, I so appreciate your careful eye throughout the editing process. The book would not be the same without you! Glenn Ramirez and Larry Pekarek, thank you so much for heartily endorsing *Generation Anxiety* and believing in this message just as much as I do. We are lucky to have such incredible mental health advocates like the two of you in publishing. Danielle Kolodkin, Andrew Gibeley, and Kevin Callahan, thank you for your creative and all-encompassing efforts to market this book so that it gets in the right hands. I'm truly grateful for your sincere dedication to this project.

I could never have done any of this alone. To the best assistant who has the most cheerful spirit I know—Jen Sandy—thank you for your unwavering light. Kelly Taylor, my publicist, thank you for believing in my message and for always seeing the value in the work that we're doing. I am so grateful that Rachel DeAlto connected us. My web designer, Sara Shepherd—you are one of the most dedicated (and fun!) women I know. How lucky am I that Upwork brought our paths together? Tiffany Morgan, thank you for always looking out for me with brand partnerships. You are a joy to work with every step of the way. Madyn Singh, thank you for making TikTok possible. I wouldn't be here without your advice . . . and hashtags. And to my dear friend, Amy Riordan, who has become one of the staunchest supporters of this book. Girl, you seriously blow me away. It's wild to think we got connected through Facebook back in the day with the Sunny Girl and Bucket List Bound adventures. Now, ten years later, we have our boys and a wonderful friendship where we are always learning from each other. I can't thank you enough for all that you've done to help promote the book. I truly could not have done this without you.

I truly love what I get to do as a psychologist and part of that is because I get to learn every day. Thank you to my clients who have opened their hearts and minds to me in the most beautiful way. I am inspired daily by your courage to lean into life. You have shown me how to live bravely and because "I've known you, I have been changed for good." Hey, what would an acknowledgments section be without a little Broadway reference from this former theater kid?

I'm also heartened by the therapists that I've been able to sit with through the years. From USC, Dr. Greg Henderson (who we will always miss), thank you for being my very first teacher in grad school who taught us to be "people first." Dr. Mary Andres, Dr. Ginger Clark, Dr. Sandy Smith, Dr. Michael Morris, Dr. Ilene Rosenstein, and the entire Rossier faculty—what an indescribable gift to learn from each of you. Thank you to my first supervisor, Joanne Weidman, for giving me the opportunity to see my very first client and for patiently guiding me as I was learning that I didn't know anything about anything as a trainee. Those were the days.

From Pepperdine, Dr. Cohen, Dr. Woo, Dr. Brunn, Dr. Bryant-Davis, Dr. Keatinge, and too many others, thank you for providing the best brain health boot camp that ever was. You taught us to always follow the science but to still come back to the heart. To my USD family, thank you for the most amazing training year of my life (in sunny San Diego, no less!). Dr. Thackray and Dr. Franklin, thank you for your gifted supervision. To my fellow interns, Carly and Hana, I count my lucky stars every day that we matched together. I hope our friendships are for life.

To my CAMPUSPEAK family—you were the first ones who believed in me as a speaker. David Stollman, thank you for this incredible opportunity that has opened so many doors. Thank you to the best agent, Monica, and David Stetter for your friendship and finesse. To my speaker family, Brittany, Rachel, Saul, Jess, Tim, Tom, Sara, Dr. Stacey, Talia, Tianna, Alex, and Dr. Christina, among so many others—I am so grateful to learn from each of you. You're all truly extraordinary.

And now to the people who have my heart. To my Grandma Joan, thank you for teaching me at a young age that "this too shall pass," and for reminding me of how family is everything. Because of you I have learned to savor the good things in life. The way you poured into my childhood with every bagel and ice cream cone—every Friday—is a gift that I will treasure forever. To my auntie Nette, thank you for being my confidante and endless supporter. You have always had my back and you're always my first call.

To my best friend, Lauren—I'm so glad that our parents took us to those swim lessons when we were babies. You are my soul sister and our relationship is one of the most cherished in my life. I can't wait for our boys to hopefully become best friends . . . #nopressure. To my nearest and dearest Abbie, Hannah, Kelly, Paige, Ailis, Lacey, Amanda, Rory, Allison, and Sarah, thank you for your beautiful friendships. I love the soulful conversations that I get to have with each of you. You are all so special to me.

To my in-laws, Russ and Debbie, thank you for encouraging me every step of the way and believing in me. I'm truly so lucky to get to call you my family. I can't wait to see the two of you become grandparents!

To my parents, words can't describe how grateful I am to be your daughter. To my dad specifically, thank you for being the funniest person I know and for always teaching me how to soak up the most of each day and have "fun, fun, fun, fun!" Thanks to you, it's gonna be a great day. To my mom, thank you for being the most mighty prayer warrior that ever was. Your love—for God, for family, for holidays, for tea party sandwiches—is so inspiring. You bring joy to everyone who knows you, but most of all, to me.

To my husband, Greg. I could write a whole book about how much I love you and the binding couldn't hold it all. When I met you on my nineteenth birthday, I knew when I saw your smile that you were someone special. Thirteen years later, I'm so glad that I still get to share my life with you. There's no one like you and my heart is entirely yours. As I told you on our wedding day, "To know you is to love you . . . and I am no exception."

To Mochi, my little Siamese cat. No one brings me more peace and happiness than you do. There is nothing like a girl and her cat, and I think we make quite the duo. You will always be my first baby.

To my son, Derek—it's wild to me that I'm writing those words. As I type this with you in my belly at thirty-three weeks pregnant, I have never been more excited to meet a person in my life. I can't believe that I get to be your mom, and I know you are going to change my heart in ways I can't even fathom. Something tells me that this will be the best adventure yet. See you soon, earth-side, my little love.

ABOUT THE AUTHOR

Dr. Lauren Cook is a licensed clinical psychologist, keynote speaker, and company consultant. She loves speaking around the country to help create more mentally healthy workplaces and schools. Dr. Cook owns a private practice, Heartship Psychological Services, where she serves individual adults, teens, and couples. Dr. Cook completed her doctorate in clinical psychology from Pepperdine University and has her master's in marriage and family therapy from the University of Southern California. She has been featured in the *New York Times*, *Forbes*, *Bustle*, and *Medium*, among other outlets. She currently lives in Los Angeles with her husband, son, and Siamese cat.

To bring Dr. Lauren to your team, visit www.drlaurencook.com.
Follow Dr. Lauren on Instagram and Tik Tok at @Dr.LaurenCook.

ENDNOTES

~~~~~~~~~~~~~~~~~~~~~~~~~~~~~~~~~~~~~~~

1. Side note: In case you're team James Cameron here and you're about to say that the doorframe wasn't buoyant enough for the two of them, I'm proud/ashamed to admit how much time I spent researching this very argument. It turns out that Jamie Hyneman and Adam Savage of *MythBusters* tested out this famous scene that has now grown quite contested. What they found is that if Rose had placed her life jacket under the doorframe, it would in fact have been buoyant enough to support both her and Jack. But honestly, who would think to do that when they're suffering from hypothermia and in the wake of a traumatic experience?

2. "Suicide Statistics," American Foundation for Suicide Prevention, https://afsp.org/suicide-statistics/.

3. "Opioid facts and statistics, " U.S. Department of Health and Human Services, December 16, 2022, https://www.hhs.gov/opioids/statistics/index.html.

4. "Marriage and Divorce," Centers for Disease Control and Prevention, March 25, 2022, https://www.cdc.gov/nchs/fastats/marriage-divorce.htm.

5. H. H. Lai, A. Rawal, B. Shen, and J. Vetter, "The Relationship Between Anxiety and Overactive Bladder or Urinary Incontinence Symptoms in the Clinical Population," *Urology* 98 (July 2016): 50–57, https://doi.org/10.1016/j.urology.2016.07.013.

6. "How Much of the Ocean Have We Explored?," National Ocean Service, February 26, 2021, https://oceanservice.noaa.gov/facts/exploration.html#:~:text=Throughout%20history%2C%20the%20ocean%20has,unmapped%2C%20unobserved%2C%20and%20unexplored.

7. "Ocean," National Geographic, May 19, 2022, https://education.nationalgeographic.org/resource/ocean.

8. M. F. Glasser and D. C. Van Essen, "Mapping Human Cortical Areas *In Vivo* Based on Myelin Content as Revealed by T1-and T2-Weighted MRI," *Journal of Neuroscience* 31, no. 32 (2011): 11597–616, https://doi.org/10.1523/JNEUROSCI.2180-11.2011.

9. R. C. Kessler, N. A. Sampson, P. Berglund, M. J. Gruber, A. Al-Hamzawi, L. Andrade, and M. A. Wilcox, "Anxious and Non-anxious Major Depressive

ENDNOTES

Disorder in the World Health Organization World Mental Health Surveys," *Epidemiology and Psychiatric Sciences* 24, no. 3 (2015): 210–26, https://doi.org/10.1017/S2045796015000189.

10. Daniel J. Siegel and Tina Payne Bryson, *The Whole-Brain Child: 12 Revolutionary Strategies to Nurture Your Child's Developing Mind* (New York: Bantam, 2012).

11. C. M. Schumann, M. D. Bauman, and D. G. Amaral, "Abnormal Structure or Function of the Amygdala Is a Common Component of Neurodevelopmental Disorders," *Neuropsychologia* 49, no. 4 (2011): 745–59, https://doi.org/10.1016/j.neuropsychologia.2010.09.028.

12. R. J. R. Blair, "Considering Anger from a Cognitive Neuroscience Perspective, *Wiley Interdisciplinary Reviews: Cognitive Science* 3, no. 1 (2012): 65–74, https://doi.org/10.1002/wcs.154.

13. J. B. Nitschke, W. Heller, P. A. Palmieri, and G. A. Miller, "Contrasting Patterns of Brain Activity in Anxious Apprehension and Anxious Arousal," *Psychophysiology* 36, no. 5 (1999): 628–37, https://doi.org/10.1111/1469-8986.3650628.

14. A. S. Engels, W. Heller, A. Mohanty, J. D. Herrington, M. T. Banich, A. G. Webb, and G. A. Miller, "Specificity of Regional Brain Activity in Anxiety Types During Emotion Processing," *Psychophysiology* 44, no. 3 (2007): 352–63, https://doi.org/10.1111/j.1469-8986.2007.00518.x.

15. "Cyclic Vomiting Syndrome," Mayo Clinic, https://www.mayoclinic.org/diseases-conditions/cyclic-vomiting-syndrome/symptoms-causes/syc-20352161.

16. D. J. Powell and W. Schlotz, "Daily Life Stress and the Cortisol Awakening Response: Testing the Anticipation Hypothesis," *PloS ONE* 7, no. 12 (2012), https://doi.org/10.1371/journal.pone.0052067.

17. G. L. Engel, "The Need for a New Medical Model: A Challenge for Biomedicine," *Science* 196, no. 4286 (1977): 129–36, https://doi.org/10.1126/science.847460.

18. F. Borrell-Carrió, A. L. Suchman, and R. M. Epstein, "The Biopsychosocial Model 25 Years Later: Principles, Practice, and Scientific Inquiry," *Annals of Family Medicine* 2, no. 6 (2004): 576–82, https://doi.org/10.1370/afm.245.

19. K. Sweeny and M. D. Dooley, "The Surprising Upsides of Worry," *Social and Personality Psychology Compass* 11, no. 4 (2017), https://doi.org/10.1111/spc3.12311.

20. Melanie Greenberg, *The Stress-Proof Brain: Master Your Emotional Response to Stress Using Mindfulness and Neuroplasticity* (Oakland, CA: New Harbinger Publications, 2017).

21. I. Ghosh, "Timeline: Key Events in U.S. History That Defined Generations," Visual Capitalist, May 7, 2021, https://www.visualcapitalist.com/timeline-of-us-events-that-defined-generations/.

22. S. Bethune, "Gen Z More Likely to Report Mental Health Concerns," *Monitor on Psychology* 50, no. 1 (2019), https://www.apa.org/monitor/2019/01/gen-z.

23. J. E. Goldstick, R. M. Cunningham, and P. M. Carter, "Current Causes of Death in Children and Adolescents in the United States," *New England Journal of Medicine* 386, no. 20 (2022): 1955–56, https://doi.org/10.1056/NEJMc2201761.

24. T. Luhby, "Many Millennials Are Worse Off Than Their Parents—a First in American History," CNN, January 11, 2020, https://www.cnn.com/2020/01/11/politics/millennials-income-stalled-upward-mobility-us/index.html.

ENDNOTES

25. K. Mathiesen, "Greta Thunberg Doesn't Want You to Talk About Her Anymore," Politico, April 28, 2022, https://www.politico.eu/article/greta-thunberg-climate -change-activism-fridays-for-future-profile-doesnt-want-you-to-talk-about-her -anymore-2022/.

26. H. R. Arkes and C. Blumer, "The Psychology of Sunk Cost," *Organizational Behavior and Human Decision Processes* 35, no. 1 (1985): 124–40, https://doi.org/10 .1016/0749-5978(85)90049-4.

27. "What Are Dissociative Disorders?," American Psychiatric Association, 2018, https://psychiatry.org/patients-families/dissociative-disorders/what-are-dissociative -disorders.

28. J. Tseng and J. Poppenk, "Brain Meta-State Transitions Demarcate Thoughts Across Task Contexts Exposing the Mental Noise of Trait Neuroticism," *Nature Communications* 11, no. 1 (2020): 1–12.

29. T. V. Maia, R. E. Cooney, and B. S. Peterson, "The Neural Bases of Obsessive-Compulsive Disorder in Children and Adults," *Development and Psychopathology* 20, no. 4 (2008): 1251–83, https://doi.org/10.1017/S0954579408000606.

30. "The U.S. Mental Health Market: $225.1 Billion in Spending in 2019: An *OPEN MINDS* Market Intelligence Report," Open Minds, May 6, 2020, https://openminds .com/intelligence-report/the-u-s-mental-health-market-225-1-billion-in-spending -in-2019-an-open-minds-market-intelligence-report/.

31. "Dissociative Disorders," in *Diagnostic and Statistical Manual of Mental Disorders*, 5th ed. (Arlington, VA: American Psychiatric Association, 2013).

32. "Who Gets OCD?," International OCD Foundation, https://iocdf.org/about-ocd /who-gets/#note-63-1.

33. P. Carey, "Common Types of OCD: Subtypes, Their Symptoms and the Best Treatment," NOCD, July 6, 2021, https://www.treatmyocd.com/education/different -types-of-ocd.

34. F. Catapano, F. Perris, M. Fabrazzo, V. Cioffi, D. Giacco, V. De Santis, and M. Maj, "Obsessive-Compulsive Disorder with Poor Insight: A Three-Year Prospective Study," *Progress in Neuro-Psychopharmacology and Biological Psychiatry* 34, no. 2 (2010): 323–30, https://doi.org/10.1016/j.pnpbp.2009.12.007.

35. S. Sauer-Zavala, J. G. Wilner, C. Cassiello-Robbins, P. Saraff, and D. Pagan, "Isolating the Effect of Opposite Action in Borderline Personality Disorder: A Laboratory-Based Alternating Treatment Design," *Behaviour Research and Therapy* 117 (2019): 79–86, https://doi.org/10.1016/j.brat.2018.10.006.

36. "Exposure and Response Prevention (ERP)," *International OCD Foundation*, https://iocdf.org/about-ocd/ocd-treatment/erp/.

37. M. M. Linehan and C. R. Wilks, "The Course and Evolution of Dialectical Behavior Therapy," *American Journal of Psychotherapy* 69, no. 2 (2015): 97–110, https:// doi.org/10.1176/appi.psychotherapy.2015.69.2.97.

38. M. Katerelos, L. L. Hawley, M. M. Antony, and R.E. McCabe, "The Exposure Hierarchy as a Measure of Progress and Efficacy in the Treatment of Social Anxiety Disorder, *Behavior Modification* 32, no. 4 (2008): 504–18, https://doi.org/10.1177 /0145445507309302.

39. C. L. Benjamin, K. A. O'Neil, S. A. Crawley, R. S. Beidas, M. Coles, and P. C. Kendall, "Patterns and Predictors of Subjective Units of Distress in Anxious Youth,"

ENDNOTES

Behavioural and Cognitive Psychotherapy 38, no. 4 (2010): 497–504, https://doi.org/10.1017/S1352465810000287.

40. "Get the Facts About Listeria," U.S. Food and Drug Administration, August 3, 2020, https://www.fda.gov/animal-veterinary/animal-health-literacy/get-facts-about-listeria.

41. A. E. Fruzzetti, "Dialectical Thinking," *Cognitive and Behavioral Practice* 29, no. 3 (2022): 567–70, https://doi.org/10.1016/j.cbpra.2022.02.011.

42. S. H. Sulzer, E. Muenchow, A. Potvin, J. Harris, and G. Gigot, "Improving Patient-centered Communication of the Borderline Personality Disorder Diagnosis," *Journal of Mental Health* 25, no. 1 (2016): 5–9, https://doi.org/10.3109/09638237.2015.1022253.

43. "Borderline Personality Disorder," National Alliance on Mental Illness, December 2017, https://www.nami.org/About-Mental-Illness/Mental-Health-Conditions/Borderline-Personality-Disorder.

44. M. Slade, S. Rennick-Egglestone, L. Blackie, J. Llewellyn-Beardsley, D. Franklin, A. Hui, and E. Deakin, "Post-traumatic Growth in Mental Health Recovery: Qualitative Study of Narratives, *BMJ Open* 9, no. 6 (2019), https://doi.org/10.1136/bmjopen-2019-029342.

45. D. Kwon, "Borderline Personality Disorder May Be Rooted in Trauma," *Scientific American*, January 1, 2022, https://www.scientificamerican.com/article/borderline-personality-disorder-may-be-rooted-in-trauma/#:~:text=Studies%20show%20that%20anywhere%20between,report%20past%20trauma%2Drelated%20experiences.

46. "Dissociative Disorders," in *Diagnostic and Statistical Manual of Mental Disorders*, 5th ed. (Arlington, VA: American Psychiatric Association, 2013).

47. C. Benjet, E. Bromet, E. G. Karam, R. C. Kessler, K. A. McLaughlin, A. M. Ruscio, and K. C. Koenen, "The Epidemiology of Traumatic Event Exposure Worldwide: Results from the World Mental Health Survey Consortium," *Psychological Medicine* 46, no. 2 (2016): 327–43, https://doi.org/10.1017/S0033291715001981.

48. Francine Shapiro, *Eye Movement Desensitization and Reprocessing (EMDR) Therapy: Basic Principles, Protocols, and Procedures* (New York: Guilford Press, 1995).

49. S. L. A. Straussner, "Micro-traumas" (presentation at the conference Trauma Through the Life Cycle from a Strengths Perspective: An International Dialogue, Hebrew University, Jerusalem, Israel, January 8, 2012).

50. Judith Lewis Herman, *Trauma and Recovery: The Aftermath of Violence from Domestic Abuse to Political Terror* (New York: Basic Books, 1997).

51. S. L. A. Straussner and A. J. Calnan, "Trauma Through the Life Cycle: A Review of Current Literature," *Clinical Social Work Journal* 42, no. 4 (2014): 323–35.

52. Sandra D. Wilson, *Hurt People Hurt People* (Grand Rapids, MI: Our Daily Bread, 2015).

53. V. Rakoff, "A Long Term Effect of the Concentration Camp Experience," *Viewpoints* 1 (1966): 17–22.

54. R. Yehuda and A. Lehrner, "Intergenerational Transmission of Trauma Effects: Putative Role of Epigenetic Mechanisms," *World Psychiatry* 17, no. 3 (2018): 243–57, https://doi.org/10.1002/wps.20568.

55. J. D. Clifton and P. Meindl, "Parents Think—Incorrectly—That Teaching Their Children That the World Is a Bad Place Is Likely Best for Them," *Journal of Positive Psychology* 17, no. 2 (2022): 182–97, https://doi.org/10.1080/17439760.2021.2016907.

ENDNOTES

56. G. N. Pandian and H. Sugiyama, "Strategies to Modulate Heritable Epigenetic Defects in Cellular Machinery: Lessons from Nature," *Pharmaceuticals* 6, no. 1 (2012): 1–24, https://doi.org/10.3390/ph6010001.

57. R. F. Afonso, I. Kraft, M. A. Aratanha, and E. H. Kozasa, "Neural Correlates of Meditation: A Review of Structural and Functional MRI Studies," *Frontiers in Bioscience-Scholar 12*, no. 1 (2020): 92–115, https://doi.org/10.2741/S542.

58. C. Lassale, G. D. Batty, A. Baghdadli, F. Jacka, A. Sánchez-Villegas, M. Kivimäki, and T. Akbaraly, "Healthy Dietary Indices and Risk of Depressive Outcomes: A Systematic Review and Meta-analysis of Observational Studies," *Molecular Psychiatry* 24, no. 7 (2019): 965–86, https://doi.org/10.1038/s41380-018-0237-8.

59. L. R. LaChance and D. Ramsey, "Antidepressant Foods: An Evidence-Based Nutrient Profiling System for Depression," *World Journal of Psychiatry* 8, no. 3 (2018): 97, https://doi.org/10.5498/wjp.v8.i3.97.

60. If you're looking for an outstanding book to help you better understand how food impacts our mental health, I highly recommend reading Dr. Uma Naidoo's book *This Is Your Brain on Food.*

61. C. A. Greene, L. Haisley, C. Wallace, and J. D. Ford, "Intergenerational Effects of Childhood Maltreatment: A Systematic Review of the Parenting Practices of Adult Survivors of Childhood Abuse, Neglect, and Violence," *Clinical Psychology Review* 80, no. 101891 (2020), https://doi.org/10.1016/j.cpr.2020.101891.

62. "Childhood Maltreatment Statistics," American Society for the Positive Care of Children, https://americanspcc.org/child-maltreatment-statistics/.

63. R. G. Tedeschi and L. G. Calhoun, "The Posttraumatic Growth Inventory: Measuring the Positive Legacy of Trauma," *Journal of Traumatic Stress* 9, no. 3 (1996): 455–71, https://doi.org/10.1007/BF02103658.

64. R. G. Tedeschi and L. G. Calhoun, "Posttraumatic Growth: Conceptual Foundations and Empirical Evidence," *Psychological Inquiry* 15, no. 1 (2004): 1–18, https://doi.org/10.1207/s15327965pli1501_01.

65. R. A. Emmons and R. Stern, "Gratitude as a Psychotherapeutic Intervention," *Journal of Clinical Psychology* 69, no. 8 (2013): 846–55, https://doi.org/10.1002/jclp.22020.

66. J. M. Kilner and R. N. Lemon, "What We Know Currently About Mirror Neurons," *Current Biology* 23, no. 23 (2013), https://doi.org/10.1016/j.cub.2013.10.051.

67. A. Bjoroy, S. Madigan, and D. Nylund, "The Practice of Therapeutic Letter Writing in Narrative Therapy," *The Handbook of Counselling Psychology* (n.p.: Sage Publications, 2016), 332–48.

68. P. Kinderman, M. Schwannauer, E. Pontin, and S. Tai, "Psychological Processes Mediate the Impact of Familial Risk, Social Circumstances and Life Events on Mental Health," *PLOS ONE* 8, no. 10 (2013), https://doi.org/10.1371/journal.pone.0076564.

69. K. Bluth and K. D. Neff, "New Frontiers in Understanding the Benefits of Self-Compassion," *Self and Identity* 17, no. 6 (2018): 605–608, https://doi.org/10.1080/15298868.2018.1508494.

70. Kristin Neff, *Self-Compassion: The Proven Power of Being Kind to Yourself* (New York: William Morrow, 2015).

71. C. Flückiger, A. C. Del Re, B. E. Wampold, and A. O. Horvath, "The Alliance in Adult Psychotherapy: A Meta-analytic Synthesis," *Psychotherapy* 55, no. 4 (2018): 316, https://doi.org/10.1037/pst0000172.

72. C. Raypole and T. J. Legg, "How to Stop People-Pleasing (and Still Be Nice)," Healthline, December 4, 2019, https://www.healthline.com/health/people -pleaser#signs.

73. S. Martin, "Signs You're a People-Pleaser," *Psychology Today*, January 4, 2021, https://www.psychologytoday.com/us/blog/conquering-codependency/202101/15 -signs-youre-people-pleaser.

74. W. Feigelman, J. Cerel, J. L. McIntosh, D. Brent, and N. Gutin, "Suicide Exposures and Bereavement Among American Adults: Evidence from the 2016 General Social Survey," *Journal of Affective Disorders* 227 (2018): 1–6, https://doi.org/10.1016 /j.jad.2017.09.056

75. "Facts and Statistics," American Association of Suicidology, 2019, https:// suicidology.org/facts-and-statistics/.

76. Side note—no hate on actual sharks. They make an incredible impact in our ecosystem, and we need them desperately. I'm using "sharks" as a metaphorical concept because, for many of us, sharks elicit a great deal of fear, and when provoked, can cause pain— just like with the examples included when people invade our personal space and time.

77. S. N. Talamas, K. I. Mavor, and D. I. Perrett, "Blinded by Beauty: Attractiveness Bias and Accurate Perceptions of Academic Performance," *PLOS ONE* 11, no. 2 (2016), https://doi.org/10.1371/journal.pone.0148284.

78. John Friel and Linda Friel, *Adult Children: The Secrets of Dysfunctional Families* (Deerfield Beach, FL: Healthcare Communications, 2010).

79. While orthorexia is not an official diagnosis in the *DSM-5*, many people struggle with this disorder, where they become obsessed with eating "healthy" food.

80. A. Kaur, A. Kaur, and G. Singla, "Rising Dysmorphia Among Adolescents: A Cause for Concern," *Journal of Family Medicine and Primary Care* 9, no. 2 (2020): 567–70, https://doi.org/10.4103/jfmpc.jfmpc_738_19.

81. J. L. Marks and A. Young, "What Is Bulimia? Symptoms, Causes, Diagnosis, Treatment, and Prevention," October 13, 2020, Everyday Health, https://www .everydayhealth.com/bulimia-nervosa/guide/.

82. J. Arcelus, A. J. Mitchell, J. Wales, and S. Nielsen, "Mortality Rates in Patients with Anorexia Nervosa and Other Eating Disorders: A Meta-analysis of 36 Studies," *Archives of General Psychiatry* 68, no. 7 (2011): 724–31, https://doi.org/10.1001 /archgenpsychiatry.2011.74.

83. STRIPED, "Social and Economic Cost of Eating Disorders in the United States," June 2020, https://www.hsph.harvard.edu/striped/report-economic-costs-of-eating -disorders/.

84. A. E. Becker, D. L. Franko, A. Speck, and D. B. Herzog, "Ethnicity and Differential Access to Care for Eating Disorder Symptoms," *International Journal of Eating Disorders* 33, no. 2 (2003): 205–12, https://doi.org/10.1002/eat.10129.

85. "Eating Disorders in LGBTQ+ Populations," National Eating Disorders Association, https://www.nationaleatingdisorders.org/learn/general-information/lgbtq.

86. L. Mulheim, and S. Gans, "Eating Disorders in Transgender People," Very-Well Mind, October 11, 2021, https://www.verywellmind.com/eating-disorders-in -transgender-people-4582520.

87. M. F. Flament, K. Henderson, A. Buchholz, N. Obeid, H. N. Nguyen, M. Birmingham, and G. Goldfield, "Weight Status and *DSM-5* Diagnoses of Eating

ENDNOTES

Disorders in Adolescents from the Community," *Journal of the American Academy of Child & Adolescent Psychiatry* 54, no. 5 (2015): 403-11, https://doi.org/10.1016/j.jaac.2015.01.020.

88. A special thank-you to the National Association of Anorexia Nervosa and Associated Disorders for providing so many of these statistics in one convenient place. If you'd like to learn more, I highly recommend going to their website at https://anad.org/.

89. S. Ulfvebrand, A. Birgegård, C. Norring, L. Högdahl, and Y. von Hausswolff-Juhlin, "Psychiatric Comorbidity in Women and Men with Eating Disorders Results from a Large Clinical Database," *Psychiatry Research* 230, no. 2 (2015): 294-99, https://doi.org/10.1016/j.psychres.2015.09.008.

90. A. Mckay, S. Moore, and W. Kubik, "Western Beauty Pressures and Their Impact on Young University Women," *International Journal of Gender and Women's Studies* 6, no. 2 (2018): 1-11, https://doi.org/10.15640/ijgws.v6n2p1.

91. E. Bruess and M. Ali, "3 Reasons why BMI Is Not an Accurate Measure of Your Health or Body Weight—and What to Use Instead," Insider, January 21, 2021, https://www.insider.com/guides/health/is-bmi-accurate#:~:text=BMI%20is%20not%20an%20accurate%20predictor%20of%20health%20because%20it,data%20from%20only%20white%20Europeans.

92. R. P. Wildman, P. Muntner, K. Reynolds, A. P. McGinn, S. Rajpathak, J. Wylie-Rosett, and M. R. Sowers, "The Obese Without Cardiometabolic Risk Factor Clustering and the Normal Weight with Cardiometabolic Risk Factor Clustering: Prevalence and Correlates of 2 Phenotypes Among the US Population (NHANES 1999-2004)," *Archives of Internal Medicine* 168, no. 15 (2008): 1617-24, https://doi.org/10.1001/archinte.168.15.1617.

93. R. Puhl and K. D. Brownell, "Bias, Discrimination, and Obesity," *Obesity Research* 9, no. 12 (2001): 788-805, https://doi.org/10.1038/oby.2001.108.

94. R. M. Puhl, T. Andreyeva, and K. D. Brownell, "Perceptions of Weight Discrimination: Prevalence and Comparison to Race and Gender Discrimination in America," *International Journal of Obesity* 32, no. 6 (2008): 992-1000, https://doi.org/10.1038/ijo.2008.22.

95. T. Osborn, " From New York to Instagram: The History of the Body Positivity Movement," BBC, https://www.bbc.co.uk/bitesize/articles/z2w7dp3#:~:text=Body%20Positivity%20begins%20with%20the,ways%20fat%20people%20were%20treated.

96. Anuschka Rees, *Beyond Beautiful: A Practical Guide to Being Happy, Confident, and You in a Looks-Obsessed World* (New York: Ten Speed Press, 2019).

97. Naomi Wolf, *The Beauty Myth: How Images of Female Beauty Are Used Against Women* (New York: William Morrow, 1991).

98. E. Aronson, B. Willerman, and J. Floyd, "The Effect of a Pratfall on Increasing Interpersonal Attractiveness," *Psychonomic Science* 4, no. 6 (1966): 227-28, https://doi.org/10.3758/BF03342263.

99. To be clear, these stereotypes are grossly overexaggerated. Someone with serious mental illness is more likely to be a victim of a crime than a perpetrator. The key predictors of violence are being young, being male-identified, and having lower socioeconomic status. In fact, you're more likely to be stabbed by someone robbing your house than by someone experiencing psychosis.

ENDNOTES

100. H. Stuart, "Violence and Mental Illness: An Overview," *World Psychiatry* 2, no. 2 (2003): 121.

101. P. M. Marzuk, "Violence, Crime, and Mental Illness: How Strong a Link? [Editorial]," *Archives of General Psychiatry* 53, no. 6 (1996): 481–86, https://doi.org/10.1001/archpsyc.1996.01830060021003.

102. A. Peterson, "Why Stereotypes About Psychosis Are Harmful," National Alliance on Mental Illness, October 8, 2020, https://www.nami.org/Blogs/NAMI-Blog/October-2020/Why-Stereotypes-About-Psychosis-Are-Harmful.

103. Larry Davidson, Janis Tondora, Martha Staeheli Lawless, Maria J. O'Connell, and Michael Rowe, *A Practical Guide to Recovery-Oriented Practice: Tools for Transforming Mental Health Care* (New York: Oxford University Press, 2009).

104. E. Ferenchick and D. Rosenthal, "Identified Patient in Family Systems Theory," in *Encyclopedia of Couple and Family Therapy* (2019), 1431–33, https://doi.org/10.1007/978-3-319-49425-8_282.

105. J. N. Ranieris, "Why Are Addiction Relapse Rates So High in Early Recovery?," Discovery Institute, July 15, 2022, https://www.discoverynj.org/addiction-relapse-rates-high-early-recovery/.

106. T. Berends, B. van Meijel, W. Nugteren, M. Deen, U. N. Danner, H. W. Hoek, and A. A. van Elburg, "Rate, Timing and Predictors of Relapse in Patients with Anorexia Nervosa Following a Relapse Prevention Program: A Cohort Study," *BMC Psychiatry* 16, no. 1 (2016): 1–7, https://doi.org/10.1186/s12888-016-1019-y.

107. C. M. Jones, R. K. Noonan, and W. M. Compton, "Prevalence and Correlates of Ever Having a Substance Use Problem and Substance Use Recovery Status Among Adults in the United States, 2018," *Drug and Alcohol Dependence* 214, no. 108169 (2020), https://doi.org/10.1016/j.drugalcdep.2020.108169.

108. J. F. Kelly, B. G. Bergman, B. B. Hoeppner, C. L. Vilsaint, and W. L. White, "Prevalence and Pathways of Recovery from Drug and Alcohol Problems in the United States Population: Implications for Practice, Research, and Policy," *Drug and Alcohol Dependence* 181 (Supplement C) (2017): 162–69, https://doi.org/10.1016/j.drugalcdep.2017.09.028.

109. D. Owens, J. Horrocks, and A. House, "Fatal and Non-fatal Repetition of Self-Harm: Systematic Review," *British Journal of Psychiatry* 181, no. 3 (2002): 193–99, https://doi.org/10.1192/bjp.181.3.193.

110. J. T. Cavanagh, A. J. Carson, M. Sharpe, and S. M. Lawrie, "Psychological Autopsy Studies of Suicide: A Systematic Review," *Psychological Medicine* 33, no. 3 (2003): 395–405, https://doi.org/10.1017/S0033291702006943.

111. M. Lim, S. Lee, and J. I. Park, "Differences Between Impulsive and Non-impulsive Suicide Attempts Among Individuals Treated in Emergency Rooms of South Korea," *Psychiatry Investigation* 13, no. 4 (2016): 389, https://doi.org/10.4306/pi.2016.13.4.389.

112. Hong Jin Jeon, Jun-Young Lee, Young Moon Lee, Jin Pyo Hong, Seung-Hee Won, Seong-Jin Cho, Jin-Yeong Kim, Sung Man Chang, Hae Woo Lee, Maeng Je Cho, "Unplanned Versus Planned Suicide Attempters, Precipitants, Methods, and an Association with Mental Disorders in a Korea-Based Community Sample," *Journal of Affective Disorders* 127, nos. 1–3 (2010): 274–280, https://doi.org/10.1016/j.jad.2010.05.027.

ENDNOTES

113. J. Ravitz, "A Widow Struggles to Make Sense of Suicide When There Were No Signs," CNN, June 22, 2018, https://www.cnn.com/2018/06/08/health/suicide-no-signs-grief.

114. M. Arain, M. Haque, L. Johal, P. Mathur, W. Nel, A. Rais, and S. Sharma, "Maturation of the Adolescent Brain," *Neuropsychiatric Disease and Treatment* 9 (2013): 449, https://doi.org/10.2147/NDT.S39776.

115. J. O. Prochaska and C. C. DiClemente, "Stages and Processes of Self-Change of Smoking: Toward an Integrative Model of Change," *Journal of Consulting and Clinical Psychology* 51, no. 3 (1983): 390, https://doi.org/10.1037/0022-006X.51.3.390.

116. N. Raihan and M. Cogburn, "Stages of Change Theory," StatPearls, 2021, https://www.statpearls.com/point-of-care/29429.

117. William R. Miller and Stephen Rollnick, *Motivational Interviewing: Helping People Change*, 3rd ed. (New York: Guilford Press, 2013).

118. C. Zhu, Y. Zhang, T. Wang, Y. Lin, J. Yu, Q. Xia, and D. M. Zhu, "Vitamin D Supplementation Improves Anxiety but Not Depression Symptoms in Patients with Vitamin D Deficiency," *Brain and Behavior* 10, no. 11 (2020), https://doi.org/10.1002/brb3.1760.

119. S. Penckofer, M. Byrn, W. Adams, M. A. Emanuele, P. Mumby, J. Kouba, and D. E. Wallis, "Vitamin D Supplementation Improves Mood in Women with Type 2 Diabetes," *Journal of Diabetes Research* (2017), https://doi.org/10.1155/2017/8232863.

120. L. Wartenberg and F. Spritzler, "Vitamin D Deficiency: Symptoms, Causes, and Treatments," Healthline, March 10, 2022, https://www.healthline.com/nutrition/vitamin-d-deficiency-symptoms#vitamin-basics.

121. O. Sizar, S. Khare, A. Goyal, P. Bansal, and A. Givler, "Vitamin D Deficiency," StatPearls, 2021, https://www.statpearls.com/point-of-care/31224.

122. N. R. Parva, S. Tadepalli, P. Singh, A. Qian, R. Joshi, H. Kandala, and P. Cheriyath, "Prevalence of Vitamin D Deficiency and Associated Risk Factors in the US Population (2011–2012)," *Cureus* 10, no. 6 (2018), https://doi.org/10.7759/cureus.2741.

123. L. E. Rhodes, A. R. Webb, H. I. Fraser, R. Kift, M. T. Durkin, D. Allan, and J. L. Berry, "Recommended Summer Sunlight Exposure Levels Can Produce Sufficient (r 20 ng ml– 1) but Not the Proposed Optimal (r 32 ng ml– 1) 25 (OH) D Levels at UK Latitudes," *Journal of Investigative Dermatology* 130, no. 5 (2010): 1411–18, https://doi.org/10.1038/jid.2009.417.

124. D. Feldman, A. V. Krishnan, and S. Swami, "Vitamin D: Biology, Actions, and Clinical Implications," in *Osteoporosis*, 4th ed., ed. Robert Marcus, David Dempster, David Feldman, and Jane Cauley (New York: Academic Press, 2013), 283–328, https://doi.org/10.1016/B978-0-12-415853-5.00013-3

125. S. L. Mumford, R. A. Garbose, K. Kim, K. Kissell, D. L. Kuhr, U. R. Omosigho, and E. F. Schisterman, "Association of Preconception Serum 25-Hydroxyvitamin D Concentrations with Livebirth and Pregnancy Loss: A Prospective Cohort Study," *Lancet: Diabetes & Endocrinology* 6, no. 9 (2018): 725–32, https://doi.org/10.1016/S2213-8587(18)30153-0.

126. A. Hunt, D. Harrington, and S. Robinson, "Vitamin B$_{12}$ Deficiency," *BMJ* 349 (2014), https://doi.org/10.1136/bmj.g5226.

ENDNOTES

127. "Thiamin: Fact Sheet for Consumers," National Institutes of Health: Office of Dietary Supplements, https://ods.od.nih.gov/factsheets/Thiamin-Consumer/.

128. "Riboflavin: Fact Sheet for Consumers," National Institutes of Health: Office of Dietary Supplements, https://ods.od.nih.gov/factsheets/Riboflavin-Consumer/.

129. "Niacin: Fact Sheet for Consumers," National Institutes of Health: Office of Dietary Supplements, https://ods.od.nih.gov/factsheets/Niacin-Consumer/.

130. D. Heitz, "Symptoms of Vitamin B Deficiencies," Healthline, August 12, 2020, https://www.healthline.com/health/symptoms-of-vitamin-b-deficiency.

131. "Folic Acid," Centers for Disease Control and Prevention, April 19, 2021, https://www.cdc.gov/ncbddd/folicacid/about.html.

132. A. Gragossian, K. Bashir, and R. Friede, "Hypomagnesemia," StatPearls, National Library of Medicine: National Center for Biotechnology Information, 2018, https://www.ncbi.nlm.nih.gov/books/NBK500003/.

133. "Magnesium: Fact Sheet for Consumers," National Institutes of Health: Office of Dietary Supplements, https://ods.od.nih.gov/factsheets/Magnesium-Consumer/.

134. R. Link and F. Sprizler, "12 Evidence-Based Health Benefits of Magnesium," Healthline, February 7, 2022, https://www.healthline.com/nutrition/magnesium-benefits.

135. E. K. Tarleton, B. Littenberg, C. D. MacLean, A. G. Kennedy, and C. Daley, "Role of Magnesium Supplementation in the Treatment of Depression: A Randomized Clinical Trial," *PLOS ONE* 12, no. 6 (2017), https://doi.org/10.1371/journal.pone.0180067.

136. D. J. White, S. De Klerk, W. Woods, S. Gondalia, C. Noonan, and A. B. Scholey, "Anti-stress, Behavioural and Magnetoencephalography Effects of an L-Theanine-Based Nutrient Drink: A Randomised, Double-Blind, Placebo-Controlled, Crossover Trial," *Nutrients* 8, no. 1 (2016): 53, https://doi.org/10.3390/nu8010053.

137. E. I. Martin, K. J. Ressler, E. Binder, and C. B. Nemeroff, "The Neurobiology of Anxiety Disorders: Brain Imaging, Genetics, and Psychoneuroendocrinology," *Psychiatric Clinics* 32, no. 3 (2009): 549–75, https://doi.org/10.1016/j.psc.2009.05.004.

138. L. Liu and G. Zhu, "Gut–Brain Axis and Mood Disorder," *Frontiers in Psychiatry* 9 (2018): 223, https://doi.org/10.3389/fpsyt.2018.00223.

139. S. Carpenter, "That Gut Feeling," *Monitor on Psychology* 43, no. 8 (2012): 50.

140. L. Liu and G. Zhu, "Gut–Brain Axis and Mood Disorder," *Frontiers in Psychiatry* 9 (2018): 223, https://doi.org/10.3389/fpsyt.2018.00223.

141. J. R. Kelly, P. J. Kennedy, J. F. Cryan, T. G. Dinan, G. Clarke, and N. P. Hyland, "Breaking Down the Barriers: The Gut Microbiome, Intestinal Permeability, and Stress-Related Psychiatric Disorders," *Frontiers in Cellular Neuroscience* (2015): 392, https://doi.org/10.3389/fncel.2015.00392.

142. J. A. Bravo, P. Forsythe, M. V. Chew, E. Escaravage, H. M. Savignac, T. G. Dinan, and J. F. Cryan, "Ingestion of Lactobacillus Strain Regulates Emotional Behavior and Central GABA Receptor Expression in a Mouse via the Vagus Nerve," *Proceedings of the National Academy of Sciences* 108, no. 38 (2011): 16050–55.

143. L. Hochwald, "9 Ways to Eat More Probiotics Every Day," Everyday Health, May 13, 2020, https://www.everydayhealth.com/diet-and-nutrition/diet/ways-eat-more-probiotics-everyday/.

144. A. H. Miller, V. Maletic, and C. L. Raison, "Inflammation and Its Discontents: The Role of Cytokines in the Pathophysiology of Major Depression," *Biological Psychiatry* 65, no. 9 (2009): 732–41, https://doi.org/10.1016/j.biopsych.2008.11.029.

145. N. G. Norwitz and U. Naidoo, "Nutrition as Metabolic Treatment for Anxiety," *Frontiers in Psychiatry* (2021): 105, https://doi.org/10.3389/fpsyt.2021.598119.

146. M. Aucoin, L. LaChance, U. Naidoo, D. Remy, T. Shekdar, N. Sayar, and K. Cooley, "Diet and Anxiety: A Scoping Review," *Nutrients* 13, no. 12 (2021): 4418, https://doi.org/10.3390/nu13124418.

147. J. Kubala and G. Tinsley, "9 Potential Intermittent Fasting Side Effects," Healthline, April 23, 2021, https://www.healthline.com/nutrition/intermittent-fasting-side-effects#Who-should-avoid-intermittent-fasting?.

148. F. Haghighatdoost, A. Feizi, A. Esmaillzadeh, N. Rashidi-Pourfard, A. H. Keshteli, H. Roohafza, and P. Adibi, "Drinking Plain Water Is Associated with Decreased Risk of Depression and Anxiety in Adults: Results from a Large Cross-Sectional Study," *World Journal of Psychiatry* 8, no. 3 (2018): 88, https://doi.org/10.5498/wjp.v8.i3.88.

149. N. Pross, A. Demazières, N. Girard, R. Barnouin, D. Metzger, A. Klein, and I. Guelinckx, "Effects of Changes in Water Intake on Mood of High and Low Drinkers," *PLOS ONE* 9, no. 4 (2014): e94754, https://doi.org/10.1371/journal.pone.0094754.

150. R. J. Stanborough and D. Weatherspoon, "Dehydration and Anxiety: How to Keep Calm and Carry On," Healthline, December 15, 2020, https://www.healthline.com/health/anxiety/dehydration-and-anxiety.

151. M. J. Aminoff, F. Boller, and D. F. Swaab, "We Spend About One-Third of Our Life Either Sleeping or Attempting to Do So," *Handbook of Clinical Neurology* 98 (2011): vii, https://doi.org/10.1016/B978-0-444-52006-7.00047-2.

152. "Sleep Deprivation Can Affect Your Mental Health," Harvard Health Publishing, August 17, 2021, https://www.health.harvard.edu/newsletter_article/sleep-and-mental-health.

153. "Healthy Sleep Habits," American Academy of Sleep Medicine, August 2020, https://sleepeducation.org/healthy-sleep/healthy-sleep-habits/.

154. "What's the Best Temperature for Sleep?," Cleveland Clinic, November 16, 2021, https://health.clevelandclinic.org/what-is-the-ideal-sleeping-temperature-for-my-bedroom/#:~:text=%E2%80%9CTypically%20it%20is%20suggested%20that,the%20stability%20of%20REM%20sleep.

155. I. M. Colrain, C. L. Nicholas, and F. C. Baker, "Alcohol and the Sleeping Brain," *Handbook of Clinical Neurology* 125 (2014): 415–31, https://doi.org/10.1016/B978-0-444-62619-6.00024-0.

156. C. Drake, T. Roehrs, J. Shambroom, and T. Roth, "Caffeine Effects on Sleep Taken 0, 3, or 6 Hours Before Going to Bed," *Journal of Clinical Sleep Medicine* 9, no. 11 (2013): 1195–1200, https://doi.org/10.5664/jcsm.3170.

157. "Exercising for Better Sleep," Johns Hopkins Medicine, https://www.hopkinsmedicine.org/health/wellness-and-prevention/exercising-for-better-sleep#:~:text=Aerobic%20exercise%20causes%20the%20body,wind%20down%2C%E2%80%9D%20she%20says.

158. J. Summer and A. Singh, "Napping: Benefits and Tips," Sleep Foundation, September 29, 2022, https://www.sleepfoundation.org/sleep-hygiene/napping#:~:text

ENDNOTES

=In%20general%2C%20the%20best%20nap,grogginess%20and%20actually
%20worsen%20sleepiness.

159. M. Hirshkowitz, K. Whiton, S. M. Albert, C. Alessi, O. Bruni, L. DonCarlos, and P. J. A. Hillard, "National Sleep Foundation's Sleep Time Duration Recommendations: Methodology and Results Summary," *Sleep Health* 1, no. 1 (2015): 40–43, https://doi.org/10.1016/j.sleh.2014.12.010.

160. "When to Seek Medical Care for Insomnia," WebMD, October 20, 2020, https://www.webmd.com/sleep-disorders/insomnia-when-to-go-to-doctor.

161. J. J. Ratey, "Can Exercise Help Treat Anxiety?," Harvard Health Publishing, October 24, 2019, https://www.health.harvard.edu/blog/can-exercise-help-treat-anxiety-2019102418096.

162. E. Anderson and G. Shivakumar, "Effects of Exercise and Physical Activity on Anxiety," *Frontiers in Psychiatry* 4 (2013): 27, https://doi.org/10.3389/fpsyt.2013.00027.

163. "Exercise for Stress and Anxiety," Anxiety & Depression Association of America, https://adaa.org/living-with-anxiety/managing-anxiety/exercise-stress-and-anxiety.

164. Michael Easter, *The Comfort Crisis: Embrace Discomfort to Reclaim Your Wild, Happy, Healthy Self* (New York: Rodale Books, 2021).

165. We featured *The Comfort Crisis* in the Brain Health Book Club. If you want to find a list of other helpful books relating to psychology and mental health, check out the list of previous reads that we've featured here: https://drlaurencook.mykajabi.com/brain-health-book-club-book-shelf.

166. "Depression and Anxiety: Exercise Eases Symptoms," Mayo Clinic, September 27, 2017, https://www.mayoclinic.org/diseases-conditions/depression/in-depth/depression-and-exercise/art-20046495#:~:text=Doing%2030%20minutes%20or%20more,time%20%E2%80%94%20may%20make%20a%20difference.

167. R. B. Ardito and D. Rabellino, "Therapeutic Alliance and Outcome of Psychotherapy: Historical Excursus, Measurements, and Prospects for Research," *Frontiers in Psychology* 2 (2011): 270, https://doi.org/10.3389/fpsyg.2011.00270.

168. "According to a New Government Survey, 38 Percent of Adults and 12 Percent of Children Use Complementary and Alternative Medicine," National Institutes of Health, December 10, 2008, https://www.nih.gov/news-events/news-releases/according-new-government-survey-38-percent-adults-12-percent-children-use-complementary-alternative-medicine.

169. P. Phutrakool and K. Pongpirul, "Acceptance and Use of Complementary and Alternative Medicine Among Medical Specialists: A 15-Year Systematic Review and Data Synthesis," *Systematic Reviews* 11, no. 1 (2022): 1–14, https://doi.org/10.1186/s13643-021-01882-4.

170. "Panic Disorder," Cleveland Clinic, https://my.clevelandclinic.org/health/diseases/4451-panic-disorder.

171. S. Breit, A. Kupferberg, G. Rogler, and G. Hasler, "Vagus Nerve as Modulator of the Gut-Brain Axis in Psychiatric and Inflammatory Disorders," *Front Psychiatry* 9 (2018): 44, https://doi.org/10.3389/fpsyt.2018.00044.

172. M. J. Tipton, N. Collier, H. Massey, J. Corbett, and M. Harper, "Cold Water Immersion: Kill or Cure?," *Experimental Physiology* 102, no. 11 (2017): 1335–55, https://doi.org/10.1113/EP086283.

173. J. Kang, A. Scholp, and J. J. Jiang, "A Review of the Physiological Effects and Mechanisms of Singing," *Journal of Voice* 32, no. 4 (2018): 390–95, https://doi.org/10.1016/j.jvoice.2017.07.008.

174. D. J. Edwards, H. Young, A. Curtis, and R. Johnston, "The Immediate Effect of Therapeutic Touch and Deep Touch Pressure on Range of Motion, Interoceptive Accuracy and Heart Rate Variability: A Randomized Controlled Trial with Moderation Analysis," *Frontiers in Integrative Neuroscience* 12, no. 41 (2018), https://doi.org/10.3389/fnint.2018.00041.

175. H. Mason, M. Vandoni, G. Debarbieri, E. Codrons, V. Ugargol, and L. Bernardi, "Cardiovascular and Respiratory Effect of Yogic Slow Breathing in the Yoga Beginner: What Is the Best Approach?," *Evidence-Based Complementary and Alternative Medicine* (2013), https://doi.org/10.1155/2013/743504.

176. L. Newhouse, "Is Crying Good for You?," Harvard Health Publishing, March 1, 2021, https://www.health.harvard.edu/blog/is-crying-good-for-you-2021030122020#:~:text=Researchers%20have%20established%20that%20crying,both%20physical%20and%20emotional%20pain.

177. At the same time, if you feel like you are always crying (often uncontrollably) and this symptom feels distressing for you, talk to a provider about it. This tearfulness can often be a biological indicator of distress and/or depression, and a biological intervention can be helpful in this case. While medication is not for everyone, I've seen several clients respond well to an antidepressant when prescribed for their tearfulness by a psychiatrist.

178. Peter A. Levine, *Healing Trauma: A Pioneering Program for Restoring the Wisdom of Your Body* (Boulder, CO: Sounds True, 2008).

179. There's a helpful video on YouTube demonstrating how this plays out with a polar bear. You can watch the video at https://www.youtube.com/watch?v=nmJDkzDMllc.

180. H. Song, F. Fang, G. Tomasson, F. K. Arnberg, D. Mataix-Cols, L. Fernández de la Cruz, Catarina Almqvist, Katja Fall, and Unnur A. Valdimarsdóttir, "Association of Stress-Related Disorders with Subsequent Autoimmune Disease, *JAMA* 319, no. 23 (2018): 2388–400, https://doi.org/10.1001/jama.2018.7028.

181. H. Song, K. Fall, F. Fang, H. Erlendsdottir, D. Lu, D. Mataix-Cols, Lorena Fernández de la Cruz, Brian M. D'Onofrio, Paul Lichtenstein, Magnús Gottfreðsson, Catarina Almqvist, and Unnur A. Valdimarsdóttir, "Stress Related Disorders and Subsequent Risk of Life Threatening Infections: Population Based Sibling Controlled Cohort Study," *BMJ* 367 (2019): l5784, https://doi.org/10.1136/bmj.l5784.

182. P. Payne, P. A. Levine, and M. A. Crane-Godreau, "Somatic Experiencing: Using Interoception and Proprioception as Core Elements of Trauma Therapy," *Frontiers in Psychology* 6 (2015): 93, https://doi.org/10.3389/fpsyg.2015.00093.

183. If you'd like to watch a helpful video to see and practice some of these somatic body exercises, here is a link: https://www.youtube.com/watch?v=xM2Z-miz3Y4.

184. "Tension & Trauma Releasing Exercises," TRE for All, Inc., https://traumaprevention.com/.

185. K. Anthony and T. J. Legg, "EFT Tapping," Healthline, September 18, 2018, https://www.healthline.com/health/eft-tapping.

186. If you're interested to learn more about how the events in our lives impact our health and somatic symptoms, take the Holmes-Rahe Life Stress Inventory. This assessment demonstrates how even generally positive events, such as getting married and reaching an outstanding personal achievement, can cause stress in the body. Here is the link: https://www.stress.org/holmes-rahe-stress-inventory.

187. M. D. Seery, R. C. Silver, E. A. Holman, W. A. Ence, and T. Q. Chu, "Expressing Thoughts and Feelings Following a Collective Trauma: Immediate Responses to 9/11 Predict Negative Outcomes in a National Sample," *Journal of Consulting and Clinical Psychology* 76, no. 4 (2008): 657, https://doi.org/10.1037/0022-006X.76.4.657.

188. M. I. Norton and F. Gino, "Rituals Alleviate Grieving for Loved Ones, Lovers, and Lotteries," *Journal of Experimental Psychology: General* 143, no. 1 (2014): 266.

189. S. M. Bögels, S. Knappe, and L. A. Clark, "Adult Separation Anxiety Disorder in *DSM-5*," *Clinical Psychology Review* 33, no. 5 (2013): 663–74, https://doi.org/10.1016/j.cpr.2013.03.006.

190. J. Feriante and B. Bernstein, "Separation Anxiety," StatPearls, 2020, https://www.ncbi.nlm.nih.gov/books/NBK560793/.

191. R. Nall and K. Kubala, "What Is Separation Anxiety Disorder in Adults?," Medical News Today, March 23, 2022, https://www.medicalnewstoday.com/articles/322070.

192. P. Hobart, "The World Is Actually Less Dangerous Than in 1990," Bustle, December 6, 2105, https://www.bustle.com/articles/127980-the-world-is-a-safer-place-now-than-it-was-25-years-ago-research-shows-which

193. S. Kitanovska, "Younger Americans Most Likely to Feel Unsafe on a Daily Basis: Poll," *Newsweek*, July 28, 2022, https://www.newsweek.com/young-americans-most-likely-feel-unsafe-daily-basis-poll-1728660.

194. "Odds of Dying," National Safety Council, 2020, https://injuryfacts.nsc.org/all-injuries/preventable-death-overview/odds-of-dying/.

195. If you'd like to learn more about these safety and injury statistics, the National Safety Council is a great website where you can access updated information: https://injuryfacts.nsc.org/.

196. "Odds of Dying," National Safety Council, 2020, https://injuryfacts.nsc.org/all-injuries/preventable-death-overview/odds-of-dying/.

197. "2021 Disasters in Numbers," United Nations Office for the Coordination of Humanitarian Affairs, April 21, 2022, https://reliefweb.int/report/world/2021-disasters-numbers.

198. C. Craighead, "As Mental Illness Rates Rise, 68% of Americans Say Social Media, News Cause Anxiety During Pandemic," *San Francisco Chronicle*, May 28, 2020, https://www.sfchronicle.com/coronavirus/article/news-social-media-cause-anxiety-during-covid-19-15300935.php.

199. "Doing Good Is Good for You Study," United Healthcare, 2017, https://newsroom.uhc.com/content/dam/newsroom/2017_VolunteerStudy_Summary_Web.pdf.

200. P. Economy, "This Is the Way You Need to Write Down Your Goals for Faster Success," *Inc.*, February 28, 2018, https://www.inc.com/peter-economy/this-is-way-you-need-to-write-down-your-goals-for-faster-success.html.